"*A Clinician's Guide to Gender Actualization: An _____ Affirming Therapy* centers the individual's gender j_____ clinicians to assist gender diverse persons in actualizing their most authentic selves. This is a needed resource that all mental health professionals working with transgender and gender diverse persons should utilize for their professional development."

Sarah Pickle, *MD, Family Medicine and Transgender Health physician*

"*A Clinician's Guide to Gender Actualization: An Approach to Gender Affirming Therapy* is an essential read for any mental health clinician working with transgender, nonbinary, or gender nonconforming individuals. Yilmazer's approach transcends traditional symptom-based methods for treating gender dysphoria by focusing on the transformative power of helping clients discover their authentic selves."

Evelyn Heflin, *clinical social worker and community leader*

"Highly recommended! Caitlin Yilmazer's work is founded on principles of reclaiming an authenticity lost to most transgender clients as they grow up unsupported in their identity. Using a self-actualization model, Yilmazer helps clients embrace their identity, shedding cultural baggage rooted in deep-seated transphobia."

Reid Vanderburgh, *retired trans therapist*

A Clinician's Guide to Gender Actualization

A Clinician's Guide to Gender Actualization provides an essential guide for mental health professionals working with gender diverse clients, delivering material that challenges clinicians to provide affirming specialized care for their clients.

Gender actualization is the social, expressive, and existential process of becoming and integrating one's authentic self through the context of gender identity, and this book introduces an effective clinical model for competent gender therapy care. Building upon the reader's foundational knowledge, chapters provide useful assessment tools, interventions, and treatment strategies to implement in their clinical practice, with accompanying personal narratives and client experiences woven throughout.

Challenging readers to explore intersectionality and the crucial awareness of their own privileges, this book is a critical read for providers working with or seeking to educate themselves regarding gender diverse clients.

Caitlin Yilmazer, LPCC-S, is a practicing counselor and the chief operating officer of Waybridge Counseling, a private practice in Cincinnati, Ohio. She has over 12 years of combined educational and clinical experience with LGBTQ+ populations. Caitlin developed the courses for LGBTQ+ and gender therapy for Xavier University. She has been a guest speaker for master's level mental health counseling courses at the University of Cincinnati, Northern Kentucky University, Union Institute, and Wright State University. Caitlin is a local presenter for gender therapy and has worked with local community resources to support Cincinnati's LGBTQ+ community, including Cincinnati Children's, Safe and Supported, ALGBTICO, and local school districts. Caitlin is primarily a practicing gender therapist and clinical supervisor at Waybridge Counseling. She continues to adjunct teach for Xavier University's mental health counseling program.

A Clinician's Guide to Gender Actualization

An Approach to Gender Affirming Therapy

Caitlin Yilmazer

Routledge
Taylor & Francis Group

NEW YORK AND LONDON

First published 2022
by Routledge
605 Third Avenue, New York, NY 10158

and by Routledge
2 Park Square, Milton Park, Abingdon, Oxon OX14 4RN

Routledge is an imprint of the Taylor & Francis Group, an informa business

Library of Congress Cataloging-in-Publication Data
Names: Yilmazer, Caitlin, author.
Title: A clinician's guide to gender actualization : an approach to
gender affirming therapy / Caitlin Yilmazer.
Description: New York, NY : Routledge, 2022. |
Includes bibliographical references and index.
Identifiers: LCCN 2021037576 (print) | LCCN 2021037577 (ebook) |
ISBN 9780367432102 (hardback) | ISBN 9780367432133 (paperback) |
ISBN 9781003001881 (ebook)
Subjects: LCSH: Gender identity disorders. | Gender identity
disorders–Treatment. | Psychotherapy.
Classification: LCC RC560.G45 Y55 2022 (print) |
LCC RC560.G45 (ebook) | DDC 616.85/83–dc23/eng/20211001
LC record available at https://lccn.loc.gov/2021037576
LC ebook record available at https://lccn.loc.gov/2021037577

ISBN: 978-0-367-43210-2 (hbk)
ISBN: 978-0-367-43213-3 (pbk)
ISBN: 978-1-003-00188-1 (ebk)

DOI: 10.4324/9781003001881

Typeset in Times New Roman
by Newgen Publishing UK

This book is dedicated to Ateş and Kaya for sharing your mother and first days of life with my writing. Many words were written with a newborn in my lap.

Contents

Acknowledgments

I have been incredibly fortunate to have experienced an outpouring of support for this book. The hundreds of clients over the years are hands down my greatest teachers and the primary contributors to my work. My peers here in Cincinnati did arduous work reading and giving me invaluable feedback to improve my writing. I want to express my gratitude for:

Yiğit, for your love and encouragement.

My family, anneciğim, for your support.

Butch, for your mentorship, friendship, and for investing in my growth since the beginning.

My Waybridge Gender Team for their passion, advocacy, and Friday meeting laughs.

Reid Vanderburgh, for your guidance and inspiration in my early clinical development.

Sarah Painer World, thank you for doing this work with me and being a part of my professional growth.

Foreword

Within a few months of opening a gender clinic at a large respected Midwest pediatric hospital, I found myself confronted by a parent in crisis shouting "I will never call you that name" in a shrill tone. The teen had presented to the clinic with depression, possible suicidal ideation and with recent disclosure of his male identity. It was 2013 and the transgender program was new to us and the community. My attending who founded the program was well versed in transgender healthcare and I was still learning the ropes, so to speak. I had confidence and competence evaluating for mental health concerns and associated risks, but I was thrust into navigating that while attending to this parents' acute crisis response to the youth's coming out. There was a complex array of emotions: fear, confusion, grief, disbelief, and possibly even embarrassment that she voiced over the hour meeting. I also immediately recognized her love for her child. This encounter heightened my awareness and insight into the impact of the role of medical and mental health providers when caring for trans individuals and their family systems.

I had always considered myself an ally for LGBTQ identified individuals but at that time I still had much to learn about allyship. I deeply believed (and still do) that all individuals should have equal access to quality healthcare and have always valued an equalist position in my personal and professional life. Therefore, accepting the role of social worker in the gender clinic was met with inspiration and hope. I immediately began my own journey of learning through professional trainings, readings, mentorship, a second master's degree and most importantly, listening to my patients/clients. While I do not have a trans experience, I have been honored to assist many on their gender journey as a resource and navigator.

At the time, the Midwest consisted of few minimally trained professionals and organizations to adequately care for trans identified youth. Youth increasingly voiced their individual expressions of gender and families often struggled to comprehend and did not know where to turn. So, we began with one 4-hour session per month dedicated to young people's gender experience. We quickly learned, "if you build it, they will come," and they did. I came across many well-intending parents who lacked a blueprint on how to respond to their child's assertion of gender, such as the parent referenced above. While the young people I work with frequently hold a clear and consistent sense of their gender, the families often are challenged by surprise, inexperience, or even lack of general direction. From these encounters, I quickly realized that supporting the trans youth meant helping the parents to reach true acceptance and this important stage can occur when gender is no longer in the forefront of the mind. However, for some, there may be many steps to take to get there.

Many parents experience emotions akin to crisis with subsequent grief and loss. In an ideal world, families would present to us as unconditionally accepting; however, since that is not always the case, we need to strive to include parents in the process without being combative or confrontational. Of critical importance is being aware of the family dynamic during the coming out and transition process; otherwise, we are doing a disservice to the patient/client. Joining with and engaging parents is crucial to the growth and development of trans and queer youth, so I advocate for accepting a family centered approach to care when applicable.

The program itself offered visibility, education and overall support for youth and their families, as well as educational training for medical and mental health professionals and evidence-based research studies. The program became a hub, with patients sometimes traveling 5–6 hours for a 30–60-minute medical appointment. Over the past eight years, the program grew from one doctor, one social worker and one half session a month to six or more full time staff with Monday–Friday availability. The patient population grew from a handful to thousands. While many families initially struggled, many came with the hope that they had finally found affirming care to help their child transition, where there previously was none. The existence of such a program decreased an important barrier: access to care, which has historically contributed to increased risks factors and mental health concerns for trans individuals. There were and still are many more barriers that need constant attention, such as: insurance/financial issues, social stigma, family acceptance, community education, clinical/medical staff being predominately cis/het, etc. It is critical that these barriers come down so specialized care can have optimal impact for trans and queer populations. While this is happening through the country, there is still much work to be done.

If you are reading this book, I hope you are embarking or expanding on your own expedition of learning. Being a trans-competent provider is not enough. Understanding the intricacies of self-actualization with gender is paramount to clinical practice. Recognizing and combating barriers, understanding that there are more than two genders, consideration for intersectionality, practicing informed consent models, and promoting gender euphoria are only a few of the necessary qualities needed for clinical practice. I hope that as time progresses, we can strive even further towards equity. Two examples of ways we can implement equity is to increase queer representation in the clinical and medical world and offer quality care that is covered by insurance. Inclusion and prioritization of professionals who have a trans and/or queer lived experience is pivotal to progressing in providing affirming medical and mental healthcare. Mental health professionals, offering informed gender affirming care, should work diligently to accept insurance and minimize cost for their patients/clients. We need insurance companies to implement inclusive policies for gender affirming care so trans individuals can have access to medically necessary interventions. Archaic policies still exist and use outdated and binary language, in essence erasing many queer and/or trans identities. Please note, these are only two examples and the list could go on and on.

Since 2019, I have worked in private practice specifically serving trans and queer identified individuals for mental health and gender affirming therapy. As a cisgender woman, I have strived to be intentional in my understanding of allyship, power, and privilege. Being an ally is not an identity or speaking for those with lived experience. Allyship is a process of uplifting and amplifying voices that are not often heard and using actions to fight for social justice and inclusion. Privilege is nuanced and allies need to know when to step back and allow for the power in others to shine. Meaningful ways to do this are through embarking on your own journey of self-actualization, furthering your understanding of that process for others and good old-fashioned listening.

As I held space with the aforementioned family and de-escalated the crisis, I worried for the young man as I sent them home. While he verbalized safety, I was unsure of how the family would continue to respond to his affirmation of gender. When they returned a few weeks later, I immediately saw his face light up as his mother, without skipping a beat, called him by his name.

Sarah Painer World, MS, MSW, LISW-S

Introduction

Gender is a deeply creative experience for humans. It presents opportunities for connection, belonging, freedom, inspiration, innovative expressions, and states of being. A self-actualized person is liberated, authentic, realistic, independent, self-loving, and feels belonging in the world. People of all genders benefit from transcending the constructs of gender to self-actualize because it makes room for the full potential of one's identity to come forward. Becoming a gender therapist has been one of the most fulfilling and transformative experiences for me, even as a cis person. It's given me an opportunity to not only pursue a specialized career path I was passionate about, but also liberate myself from rigid expectations surrounding gender. In actualizing my own gender identity as a core aspect of who I am and how I interact with the world, I have been able to expand my fulfillment and overall quality of life within my social relationships, family, marriage dynamics, career, self-expression, medical advocacy, sense of self and identity, and interaction with day to day society.

That said, much of my self-enlightenment is nurtured by my privilege of being cisgender. Gender diverse individuals are not granted the ability to self-actualize because of significant oppressive systems that leave trans folx abandoned and punished for simply being authentic. Gender is inherently both healing and oppressive, especially so for trans people. Healing is found through affirmation of gender and being seen and embraced for the authentic self. But in order to feel affirmed, there's immense pressure to subscribe to a binary gender and its rigid rules. For binary trans folx, this subscription demands strict conformity which can stifle one's freedom and creativity. That experience presents a barrier. As a cis woman, I can push and bend boundaries around my gender because from day one there has been unwavering social affirmation that has provided me a privilege of being seen for who I am. When someone is seen and affirmed, it's a door that opens to self-actualization. This affirmation is granted to cis people from birth, leaving them without the immense challenges and obstacles of navigating a world of rejection and oppression.

The concept of gender actualization was born from a brainstorming session with my friend and mentor who was my clinical supervisor for three years. Butch and I were writing an article on transitioning families,

DOI: 10.4324/9781003001881-1

combining his expertise in the systemic model and my specialty in gender therapy. We never got around to publishing it, so I included our work in a chapter in this book. He asked me to explain my model, my clinical approach for gender therapy, and asked me to explore with him what the term transition entailed. We both found the term to be too limiting and simplistic in writing about the deeply complex and personal experience that comes with transitioning. I explained the intricate process, the deconstruction and reconstruction of every facet of life that was built around an identity assigned to the person. Transition is about reclaiming authenticity—the privilege cisgender people are born with. Days later, he came to me and said my description reminded him of the concept of Abraham Maslow's self-actualization, and thus the term for gender actualization was born.

If I were to simplify my perspective of gender therapy, it is leading the client towards actualizing the self through the context of gender. The basis of clinical work in the mental health field is rooted in helping our clients actualize themselves, but the context always changes. It's always about the identities of our clients and how various circumstances and experiences are defining them. My approach is less about what it is like to be trans, as each experience is unique and different and out of my ability to comprehend as cisgender. It's about self-actualization through the context of gender. My "model" or approach to gender therapy is eclectic. I use interventions and a variety of therapeutic orientations ranging from, but not limited to, attachment, Satir practices, systemic approaches, cognitive behavioral therapy (CBT), strengths-based practices, family of origin work, affirmative therapy, shame reduction for internalized stigma, narrative therapy, and parts work. This method supports flexibility for the diverse orientations of clinicians working with this population.

Another aspect of my personal framework for gender therapy is to provide a more concrete clinical approach to working with gender diversity. This not only helps clinicians, since we need our procedures to be effective clinicians, but I've found it helps many clients feel more grounded in their own actualizing process. Actualizing one's gender is a completely vague concept with minimal clear definitions, protocol, and absolutely zero guarantees for what the outcome will look like. Having some sort of structured outline that informs clinical approach isn't only ethically expected of clinicians for best practice, it provides our clients a feeling of security within the therapeutic space. While having some sort of model in our practice, it's also important to subscribe to the ambiguity of gender and applying it to clinical work, otherwise we'd be perpetuating pathological binary stereotypes associated with trans people. Being comfortable with ambiguity, and even mystery, is a necessary part of the deeply complex processing work conducted in talk therapy with gender clients.

I am adding more cisgender opinion to the mix of trans education and it reminds me to be extremely aware and cautious about the impact I might have on clinical discourse on gender therapy. The same as every therapist with certain privileges that have impact on clients of marginalized groups they work with. I feel an immense pressure to honor my clients; they have given me the greatest gift of their stories and they are my best teachers. Their voices inspired and informed every page of this book. I have blind spots and will continue to learn them as long as I do this work. Being white, straight, and cis doesn't leave a lot of room for firsthand marginalization. Being a woman gives me cognitive empathy, but not much direct empathic experience for gender diversity. Though we are seeing advancement, there is an extreme lack of trans mental health professionals available to provide appropriate representation for the diversity of clientele. With this lack of trans clinicians, and support for them, their rightful contributions to discourse and education of gender therapy are often left out. This is important to keep in mind when specializing in gender therapy because gender therapists should make very conscious efforts to seek education from trans professionals.

My hopes in writing this book is to contribute what I can as a clinician to the practice of gender therapy. I am sharing knowledge gained from working with hundreds of gender therapy clients, hours of formal education, years of supervision and consultations with national experts, involvement in my local trans community, and experience in training and education on the subject in Cincinnati. While there are some aspects of gender therapy that are standard for professionals, I am optimistic I can offer more to practitioners dedicated to this specialty.

1 Tales of the Well-Intended Gatekeeper

The counseling profession demands quality care for our ever-diversifying world. Not only do our clients expect us to be informed clinicians, but so do our peers. The clinical community is systemic. Clinicians rely on the qualifications of one another to provide comprehensive care for clients. Counselors depend on the competence of the clinicians they are referring to, and we refer to one another for several reasons: need of higher level of care, specific or specialized treatment, client overflow, or additional resources are indicated. Just like any specialized population, working with the LGBTQ+ and trans populations requires specific clinical education, unique treatment approaches, and ongoing stewardship. Unfortunately, this courtesy has been denied to trans and LGBTQ+ communities for too long because many medical and mental health professionals have ignored adjusting their practice approaches to meet the specific treatment needs.

Very recently, the clinical community began integrating LGBTQ+ care regularly into trainings and workshops, primarily since it is considered a "hot topic." This change is a victory; it's an indicator of growth. Now, we have a sea of generally informed "LGBTQ+ friendly" therapists and allies flooding the scene, but clients are still struggling to receive effective care. This book is intended as a contribution to the next step, encouraging clinicians to specialize in trans counseling, just as any other population we are expected to specialize in. Trans populations have very specific and unique treatment needs and clinicians should be expected to undergo appropriate training just as any other counseling population. Failure to do this runs the risk of "gatekeeping."

The term "gatekeeper" is used by the LGBTQ+ community to describe individuals in helping fields who are in a position of power and intentionally or unintentionally abuse that authority to delay or block a person's access to resources. A gatekeeper controls the "gate" and is the one who has permission to pass through it. Gatekeepers are not always mental health clinicians, they are doctors, lawyers, teachers, parents, managers, peers, and any other person who has authority over another's ability to access needs. For the sake of better understanding, it's a similar concept to privilege. Societal structure is set up in a way that the actions of people with privilege

DOI: 10.4324/9781003001881-2

(and privilege bestows power) impact marginalized populations who are systematically stuck, at the mercy of the privileged authority.

Though gatekeeping has a lot of negative connotations, gatekeeping behavior (most of the time) stems from the positive intention of holding space and boundaries that were ultimately intended to be healthy for all involved. For example, certain standards of care were intended to give a framework for providers to work with and help trans populations while also working within the laws, ethics, and professional demands of their license. As these standards became societally outdated, providers still following them could unintentionally become gatekeepers, unaware of the impact this had on their clients.

Let's briefly examine standards of care, another loaded topic. Standards of care are inherently gatekeeping, but clinicians are not at the top tier assigning and executing these rules. They are mere enforcers of these orders just like every other provider working with trans populations. Clinicians and medical providers follow these standards because they have to in order to get insurance companies to cover medically necessary interventions for clients and patients. So doesn't this really make us all gatekeepers? Yes, it does. So let's work together to lessen the blow of this reality for the populations we serve. Clinicians who are well-informed and seasoned with trans populations are better able to navigate the structures in place to support and advocate for the dignity of our clients as they journey through the deeply complex process of gender actualization and transition.

There are core differences between the trans-friendly and trans-specialized clinicians. This chapter is not intended to be attacking or accusatory of the trans-friendly therapists, rather challenge these professionals to continue seeking growth to better serve their clients—to help them understand their impact. At one time or another, because of our humanity, clinicians will be or have been gatekeepers out of naivety, not maliciousness. There is always a learning curve that comes with mastering a skill or expertise. I'm sure I have been someone else's gatekeeper unknowingly along my own journey. Taking the time to listen to marginalized populations, mindfully internalize the information, and grow is our responsibility as helpers—especially those of us who are placed in a position of authority. Taking a stance of humbleness and vulnerability, while difficult, is necessary to inspire professional and interpersonal growth.

I have collected some stories, or tales, depicting gatekeeping behaviors either peers, clients, or I have encountered. These vignettes are intended to increase mindfulness and awareness of the true impact we can have unintentionally on the clients we have vowed to help and serve.

The Outdated Gatekeeper

My first experience connecting with another trans-informed mental health professional was disappointing. This clinician was seasoned and well-known in the LGBTQ+ community, a local pioneer. I'm certain at one time, they were *the* progressive professional of the community, and I'm sure they are passionate about their work and helping the community. During our initial meeting, I was first handed a copy of the Harry Benjamin Standards of Care, which is an outdated document that has been replaced by World Professional Association for Transgender Health (WPATH) Standards of Care. I was also handed a clinical assessment packet for the purpose of collecting extensive sexual histories of clients. This clinician informed me they refuse to provide letters of medically necessary Hormone Replacement Therapy (HRT) until their clients present themselves as their intended gender, or "dress" for them, in sessions. They strictly followed the Harry Benjamin Standards of Care which enforced outdated standards that could be considered somewhat cruel to clients today. This professional uses an extensive sexual history assessment with all trans clients, leading me to wonder how appropriate and relevant the assessment was for gender therapy. Lastly, I asked a question about the assessment process for an HRT letter, and this professional cautioned me about possible comorbid symptoms of Dissociated Identity Disorder (DID) and that I should be incredibly cautious during my diagnostic assessment process for gender therapy. Knowing what I know now, it is actually common practice for gender therapy clients to conceptualize and process their gender identity by projecting their personas—similar, but not the same, as ED with eating disorder treatment, or like parts work. To normalize the stigma of comorbidity between these two diagnoses is troubling and further perpetuates the pathological ideas about gender identity. Clinicians providing gender therapy need to continue their education and actively seek ongoing training, supervision or peer consultation, and resources to stay up to date.

The Liability Gatekeeper

Unfortunately, I do not have an isolated case or single story about this type of gatekeeper. I have received countless phone calls and emails from potential clients asking me about my standards for providing letters for HRT and Gender Affirming Surgery (GAS) consultation—many the result of horrible experiences with liability gatekeepers. Liability gatekeepers come from the well-intentioned place of protecting their license, which is a legitimate priority for all clinicians. Due to lack of training or competence, these clinicians continue to see trans clients without appropriate referral or supervision for a multitude of reasons: a need for clients because of low client load, desire to help and provide treatment because they are LGBTQ+ allies, or because they do not know who else to refer to. Once trans clients progress in their process of actualization and decide they want to consult with a provider about HRT, these gatekeepers are faced with the consequence of keeping these clients without referring them to a more appropriate clinician or becoming more informed themselves. The end result is that clients wind up spending hundreds of dollars for services under the impression that the clinician would provide a letter, and the clinician tells them it is neither their policy nor practice to do so. This delays the client's process of transition by weeks or months. Transition is expensive, and this type of experience depletes necessary funds. Because most medical HRT providers follow WPATH standards and resist informed consent practice, clients must have this letter with their diagnoses of gender dysphoria in order to start HRT treatment. These individuals are then forced to find a new therapist and start all over again. This takes a personal and financial toll on a trans person's transition process. Essentially, the liability gatekeeper feels they are not competent enough to provide the HRT letter, and to avoid any potential risk or liability to their license, they refuse to give it. At the very least, if these clinicians can't or won't refer to a gender therapist, I encourage to at the very least, to get a copy of WPATH Standards of Care so that they feel confident enough to write HRT letters.

The Ally Only Gatekeeper

The Ally Only Gatekeeper embodies the clinician who might pat themselves on the back once the letter for HRT is provided, and then call it a day. These gatekeepers often pride themselves in knowing the 101 knowledge about gender identities and using their ally powers to help save the day. Another presentation of this gatekeeper is a person who may be very well informed on the ins and outs of the LGBTQ+ and gender populations but lack additional experience or skills to do deeper therapeutic work. Though this can be great practice for the clients who are just seeking their letter (like the clients who suffered above with the liability gatekeeper), there are many people who would benefit from gender therapy as they progress towards gender actualization. Once ongoing treatment is indicated, the Ally Only Gatekeeper often falls short due to lack of training, ongoing self-education, or appropriate supervision or consultation. I've received reports from clients that these gatekeepers will often make the "I'm not very informed on these issues, I do not know how to help you with that" when faced with subjects specific to gender therapy. These gatekeepers are a great step towards progress and have positive intentions to help; however, they fall short in clinical expertise to practice gender therapy. Clients are then forced to start all over with a new therapist when they were initially under the impression that their therapist would be able to help them through the whole process. Clinicians like this should be transparent from the start, mentioning in their clinical impression reflection after the assessment that they may refer out if more in-depth gender therapy is indicated. Or they could work towards specialization.

I am aware that I was unknowingly some form of a gatekeeper when first starting as a counselor. When I was just getting started as a counselor, I had a strong educational background in LGBTQ+ issues. This was marketable for the places I worked, so I often got referrals for these cases. Cincinnati, at the time, was just starting to create more LGBTQ+ programs, but there was an enormous and glaring lack of gender therapists. Because of these factors, I was bombarded with trans-identified client referrals. Knowing that my competence was just getting started, I consulted with my clinical supervisor at the time for what to do to best meet this demand. He encouraged me to seek out an international expert to consult and have regular supervision with, engage in active research and set annual training goals, and to write. Writing is a great way to build specialty as it forces intensive self-education. I did these things while working in tandem with clients. For a brief stint of time, I was this gatekeeper. Because everyone has to start somewhere, I encourage anyone who acknowledges they are in this boat to just simply continue advancing.

The Experimental Gatekeeper

The Experimental Gatekeeper encourages clients to experiment with stereotypical myths of the trans community. One time a client admitted to me that she regressed for six months in her transition process because of an experience with her previous therapist. She told me that though her previous therapist was well-intentioned, they encouraged her to attend some local drag shows so she could "see what it's like." This was a bold suggestion for the therapist to make, and while apparently well-intentioned, this microaggression scared my client into regression, fearing that her transition process would be yet another performance she would be forced to live. Clinicians should actively work on deconstructing their own ideas about gender diversity in order to work with these populations. This clinician probably thought performers of drag are transgender or that the shows might be welcoming for their trans clients. However, in making such generalizations, the client felt reduced to a certain dramatized performance of femininity. Making her feel the therapist saw her identity as something to be performed rather than lived.

There's an ongoing debate on whether drag performers are adopted under the trans umbrella. Drag performers do not always identify as trans, while others do. Drag is a performance, but it also expects its performers to exude their own personal expansive gender experiences; this can qualify the royalties of drag to identify under the trans umbrella. There's even more debate on the impact drag practice has on the present trans community, but it is most times currently accepted and adored due to the culturally rich and deep history drag and the ballroom scene have given to the LGBTQ+ and trans community. Drag and ball communities have contributed significantly to the gay liberation movement while providing a space of creative freedom for LGBTQ+ folx.

The Tolerating Gatekeeper

The Tolerating Gatekeeper is essentially what the title sounds like. They tolerate, while not really accepting or supporting trans clients, by separating personal values from work. Though this ability can appear admiral, does this cognitive dissonance really create a safe space? Whether we try to differentiate it, our personal values do inform and guide our work. For example, I've heard of counselors who have worked with gay clients to suppress sexuality because it was the client's directly stated goal. For clinicians with an affirming lens, this would have been addressed immediately in the first session as something that won't be done. It would be communicated that it is not ethical to provide this type of treatment since sexuality is an innate unchanging aspect of who a person is. I would challenge these clinicians with an affirming lens and normalize and integrate sexuality into the client's life rather than offer to help repress it; it ventures into a strange gray area of client's goals vs. conversion therapy. Though well-intentioned (as most gatekeepers), personal values do find ways to impact our work as clinicians whether we like it or not. It's the responsibility of the clinician working with LGBTQ+ and trans clients to challenge and change any conflicting values.

The Detective Gatekeeper

I was once contacted by a medical HRT provider who was seeking further information about the assessment and treatment of a former client of mine. I had provided a letter verifying this client's diagnosis and treatment history, encouraging this client and the HRT doctor to consult about possible HRT intervention. This provider was investigating the legitimacy of the client's need for HRT intervention because the client came to her appointment with incongruent gender expression. This client identified as a woman and came to her HRT appointment in masculine presentation, including facial hair, which perplexed the doctor. This provider was obviously not aware of the many possibilities as to why this situation can occur, including that it is common for transgender individuals to start HRT long before their expressive and social transition begins. Let alone understanding the entire spectrum of gender identity that could explain situations such as these occurring. The Detective Gatekeeper relies on other professionals to provide them with sufficient evidence to open the gate to accommodate their lack of knowledge and competency. These gatekeepers essentially want to defer as much liability in opening the gate due on others due to their own lack of education and training. Liability and detective gatekeepers can be co-occurring!

The Paid Friend Gatekeeper

The Paid Friend Gatekeeper is a familiar character within all clinical populations. This professional will continue to see clients even when they are no longer serving the best interest of the client, usually under the pressure of the client–provider rapport. Pressure can come from the client who is hesitant to move on due to connection to their provider, or it can stem from the clinician who believes the therapeutic rapport is enough. I had a client who spent two years with another clinician, describing to me it was a "paid friend" type of relationship that led them nowhere in gender actualizing. After two years, this clinician finally decided to tell the client that they are not competent enough to help them any longer with their gender identity. For two years this clinician was aware of the gender identity problems; yet they decided to treat depression and allow rapport-type treatment to continue with minimal progress. During this large window of time, a referral could have been made or the clinician could have developed competency. Clinicians sometimes feel pressured by their clients (and the relationship rapport) to continue seeing them even when a referral is warranted. Clients of Paid Friend Gatekeepers have good rapport with their clinician which encourages them to stay in treatment even when they are not getting what they need. Sometimes clients will deny their own best interest and refuse a referral because they are afraid they won't like a new therapist as much as the Paid Friend. These are the tough times as a clinician because it's our duty to do the tricky process of enforcing a proper referral while also preparing and transitioning the client in their own readiness.

The "Educate Me" Gatekeeper

A common phrase I hear from clinicians with little experience in LGBTQ+ and trans counseling is "the client can educate me on their experience." This clinician is often implying that they will rely on the client to tell them what the terminology means, what gender dysphoria is like, and really every nook and cranny about the transition process. I cannot stress enough how exhausting this is for trans folx. These clients are coming to treatment for guidance, not the other way around. It is the duty of the mental health provider to be informed enough to do the deeply complex and unique work with clients. Gender therapy is a complicated dance that looks different for every client. If the clinician is not experienced with the material to begin with, the client misses out on the opportunity to do important processing work. Not to mention that most marginalized populations are absolutely fatigued by the lack of initiative of the privileged to educate themselves from time to time. Yes, the most crucial form of learning is through information sharing and dialogue, but in the clinical context where clients are seeking our knowledge, this type of exchange just isn't professional. Counselors often rely on this skill, learning from our clients, because we are expected by our licensure standards to adapt to all sorts of clients and still give quality treatment. We do see a variety of clinical issues and are always on our toes because once we think we've seen it all, we get something new. We are taught in our education how to adapt and accommodate clients while ensuring we provide good care, so the "Educate Me" Gatekeeper is a product of the basic clinical expectations of mental health providers.

Don't get me wrong, the most of my learned experiences with this population came from my clients. My clients continue to keep me up to date, taught me almost everything I know, and continue to challenge my cisgender-influenced world views that I didn't even know existed. My clients are the most influential and richest resource of knowledge I have and I wouldn't be writing this book without their bravery and willingness to share their stories with me. That said, it takes initiative on my part to do the reading, watching media, paying for consultation with national experts, attending trainings, and participate in social media lurking to ensure my clients are minimally impacted by anything I lack.

Microaggressions

There is something these stories all have in common, a theme around microaggressions. Chester M. Pierce, MD is known for first coining the term microaggressions (in the 1970s) to describe the subtle slights or insults he observed black Americans endure by non-black Americans as a result of marginalization. The term has greatly expanded and is now common language when working within the psychology and sociology fields. It's also a frequent topic of discussion when addressing social justice and societal oppression. Microaggressions are the intentional or unintentional, nonverbal or verbal, subtle or not-so-subtle communication of insults, dismissals, hostility, threats, derogatory slights, and other negative messages that specifically target a person based on their membership in a marginalized group. These types of behaviors are different from overt or direct aggressions (a macroaggression) because most of the time the perpetrator does not consciously carry intent to harm and unknowingly fosters the discrimination (Sue, 2010).

Clients take emotional risks to be open and vulnerable with their therapist. When they experience a microaggression in what is supposed to be a safe place, it can quickly erode trust and encourage a negative belief system surrounding their identity. Trust ruptures in the therapeutic relationship are bound to happen with every population because clinicians are human. A part of being human is committing to being a forever student, and clinicians are not above this. Clinicians are constantly learning and growing and with the added pressure of being artistic linguists and creatively navigating every session by sheer improv skills, we are bound to make slips. Some other examples of microaggressions in sessions include:

Redirecting Sessions to Client's Gender Identity or Transition When Client Has Not Expressed Its Relevance

Some clients come to sessions seeking consultation or treatment surrounding specific needs not related to transition. Some gender therapists, like myself, might argue that it's almost impossible not to address gender identity even in post-transition since gender actualization is lifelong because society has made it impossible to escape. Our culture is the sole culprit for extending this process for trans folx. However, there are circumstances where a client is coming to consult about very specific matters. In these cases, gender is not for the clinician to prioritize and address. If a clinician is too eager or acting out of curiosity, it can cause internalized shame or inadvertently cause the client to feel dehumanized. It can also take away from the unique experiences of the client to overly normalize everything to gender, as a client wants to be seen as an individual and not a group.

Making Statements such as "You Look Like a Woman" or "You Pass"

This subtly assigns the mental health professional as the authority (or dare I say gatekeeper?) of cisgender beauty standards. Let's break this down. Our culture has assigned standards of gender expression that are acceptable, and these standards are rooted in rigid binary and misogynistic ideas of what is considered attractive for men and women. Folx of binary or nonbinary gender identities may not fall into these limiting boxes; even most cisgender people do not live up to these impossible standards. This isn't to say that clinicians will never face a client who asks them if they "pass." As I touched in Introduction on use of this term, I want to note again that I completely avoid this term since it indicates that the person is somehow being deceptive and assigns success and failure. Cisgender clinicians should especially avoid taking this role of "gender police" because it creates an uncomfortable power dynamic, since the cisgender identity carries privilege; and that privilege has the ability to perpetuate discrimination. If asked by a client, I openly explain to them that I'm uncomfortable with this role due to my privilege and sometimes this leads to a therapeutic discussion. This doesn't necessarily mean compliments are off the table; it just needs to be a well-thought out and conscious action that doesn't support the abuse of power and privilege.

Dismissing or Brushing off Transgressions that Occur in Sessions

Some offenses clinicians might commit against trans clients are: misgendering, using assigned name at birth (some call *dead-naming*), making cis and straight assumptions about the client, use of dehumanizing or outdated language, and making statements that minimize the legitimacy of the client's gender identity. To be able to simply brush off any of these experiences is a cis privilege and cannot be expected of our clients who are taking the emotional and vulnerable risk of inviting the therapist into their world. The same applies to all marginalized populations, specifically black, indigenous, and people of color (BIPOC) who are disenfranchised and oppressed as a result of white privilege. Some mental health providers are under the belief system that not all clinical ruptures need to be addressed. I've heard professionals take the defensive stance that in order for a person to build resilience in the imperfect nature of the world, they need to learn to brush off a mistake made by the therapist; this is coming from the assumption that the infractions are so insignificant that they should be dismissed. The trans and LGBTQ+ community are already extremely resilient due to the astounding amounts of courage it takes to exist in a society that treats these individuals as pathological outsiders. These clients do not need to reexperience the trauma they face daily from the outside world inside the therapeutic setting. There will always be accidental transgressions in this line of work, and it's the duty of the professional to take accountability for the safe place that's being promised.

I had been working with a client for six months before he was comfortable enough for me to use his identified name and pronouns. When he first came to therapy, he wanted me to use his assigned name and pronouns at birth because he was "just not there yet." He was uncomfortable initially because he was just starting his gender actualization process and he needed time to adjust to the change. After six months, he gave me his names and pronouns to use as he began transition and felt ready. During an email exchange regarding rescheduling an appointment, I mindlessly and accidentally addressed him incorrectly because I was used to using his assigned name at birth. Immediately after I sent the email I was overcome with shame and embarrassment. I promptly sent an apology. Later that day he emailed me the response: "It's okay, I'm getting used to the name too." I followed up with him in our next session, prepared to work on mending a trust rupture, but he was adamant that he had not been very impacted by this event because he was prepared for this process to have some messy moments.

Mending Clinical Ruptures

I share this story often with students and colleagues to prepare them for the inevitable clinical ruptures. A clinical rupture can be an acute or building tension that contributes to the breakdown of the therapeutic team, or the relationship between therapist and client. Clinical ruptures in the therapeutic relationship happen across the wide range of clients that clinicians see, and the trans and LGBTQ+ populations have higher risk of these ruptures occurring. I refer to a subcategory of clinical ruptures as *trust ruptures*, primarily for this population because trust is absolutely necessary in the therapeutic alliance when working with gender diverse clients. Trust is often gained over several sessions and extensive rapport building. It is built within the therapeutic relationship because clients are often working through interpersonal issues within the context of treatment or in their relationship with their therapist. Outside of the office, these individuals are routinely facing violence, prejudice, oppression, microaggressions, gatekeeping, family and social rejection, bullying, and loss due to their identity. Preservation of trust creates resilience, so clinicians should be mindful of this dynamic in therapy. Unintentional negative events that clients experience with their clinician foster the internalized transphobia and shame the individual has suffered for simply existing.

The therapeutic alliance is such a powerful relationship that it is a primary indicator of therapy outcomes. Conversely, poor therapeutic alliances consisting of clinical ruptures negatively impact outcomes for treatment and have a direct correlation on predicting early termination or drop out. Two types of ruptures are withdrawal and confrontation ruptures. Withdrawal ruptures describe the distancing or avoidant-type behaviors because of client dissatisfaction or discontent. Confrontation ruptures are when the client confronts the clinician with negative feelings about the therapist or treatment. According to a study by Eubanks, Burckell, and Goldfried (2018), there are two very effective ways to manage clinical ruptures. The first is rupture-bond, which is to explore with clients the impact or experience they had with the rupture. The second is to validate, or acknowledge, the client's perspective about the rupture. Other effective interventions include information gathering, coping strategies, and focus on emotional experience. Of all these interventions, clinicians were unable to rate a consistently effective way to manage confrontation ruptures, as professionals struggle most with these types of ruptures (Eubanks, Burckell, & Goldfried, 2018).

First and foremost, when a clinician makes a mistake, they should promptly issue a correction. Most clients, and trans individuals in general, carry anxiety surrounding correcting others. By correcting ourselves, we are taking charge of the rupture that occurred and removing the burden from the client to address it. Doing so also informs the client that we are aware of the rupture. Clinicians sometimes fail to do this out of personal feelings that arise with the rupture—we sometimes freeze. Additional findings from Eubanks, Burckell, and Goldfried (2018) support that therapists who are more impacted by internal feelings of guilt and shame, which lead to feelings of incompetence, experience more impairment in their ability to manage ruptures effectively. If and when this happens, it's important to process the rupture with a peer or supervisor so that the most effective course of action can take place, unclouded by therapist shame. Being aware of our own emotional reactions, and taking responsibility for them, unburdens clients from managing our feelings and increases success for repairing trust and clinical ruptures.

To further address the clinical or trust rupture, clinicians should then explore the impact and experiences the client had to the rupture, and respond with empathy, compassion, and validation. The level of personal disclosure is up to the clinician and their professional approach and orientation. I strongly suggest practicing mindfulness about how much disclosure is shared in order to avoid client feeling responsible for clinician's emotions. Clinical ruptures are bound to happen with all populations, and gender therapists should be prepared for these moments to happen. They happen to even the most experienced and knowledgeable mental health providers.

In order to be a highly effective gender therapist, ongoing personal reflection and self-awareness is a key. Our professional identities are constantly expanding and changing, as we undergo our own unique stages of development. Understanding our personal strengths and weaknesses is an important part of seeking growth opportunities, and we are trained to use our own internal processes to inform our clinical actions and pursuits. If a clinician is working with a population without proper training and supervision, there is risk of negative consequences for clients and even the potential for harm. The goal of this chapter is to encourage clinicians to step in or step out, preferably step in. By stepping in, the clinician is committing to expansion through education, training, dedication, advocacy, consultation, and a level of immersion by connecting to the LGBTQ+ and trans communities. If the clinician opts to step out, this means recognizing that their specific expertise or clinical contributions are better suited for other populations. Clinicians stepping out are committed to providing accurate and helpful resources for trans clients who find them.

Reflection Questions for Clinicians

1   How are you currently a gatekeeper? What steps can you take to ensure clients are not inadvertently being harmed by your gatekeeping?
2   Identify a microaggression that you have committed. How did you/or should have mended this rupture? If you cannot identify one, think of a plausible scenario in which you could commit a microaggression in session, and how can you mend it?
3   How do you feel about referring (when able to) clients when they need specialized care you are not experienced enough in? If you cannot refer, what steps should you take as a clinician?

References

Eubanks, C. F., Burckell, L. A., & Goldfried, M. R. (2018). Clinical consensus strategies to repair ruptures in the therapeutic alliance. *Journal of Psychotherapy Integration*, 28(1), 60–76. doi:10.1037/int0000097

Sue, D. W. (2010). *Microaggressions and marginality: manifestation, dynamics, and impact*. Hoboken, NJ: Wiley.

2 Cultural Humility

Cultural humility and competency are necessary foundations for any professional in the mental health field. Awareness of the intersectionality of the privileges that impact our own perceptions and world view is critical in working with clients. In the human services fields, we must practice mindful self-reflection when working with people from all walks of life. Manifesting self-awareness is a process of addressing internalized biases, prejudices, and assumptions about the world used to make connections and fuel perceptions. This process ultimately instills a sense of accountability and responsibility, which fuels change and action within the individual. It motivates the person to influence change through personal behavior and hopefully work towards larger scale changes.

In this chapter I will break down a few important nuggets that are critical when working with marginalized populations, primarily trans individuals. Our brains are still not capable of not forming prejudice, so I will first break down the cognitive process of prejudice. It's a basic cognitive process used for survival, and acknowledging this truth is key in self-awareness and is necessary for systemic change. Addressing prejudice also aids in the deconstruction of the binary social categorization of gender. I will also address privilege, intersectionality, and the importance of affirming and expansive language. These are all necessary to the foundation a clinician must be aware of when working with gender populations.

Unconscious bias is the automatic and unconscious stereotyping pulled from a reservoir of learned prejudice. Typically, these beliefs are about persons outside of one's own social group and the judgments formed lack evidence or support. At least in this time, humans are not capable of being free of prejudice. It's deeply ingrained and sewn into culture in some form or another, and humans are systematically programed to include these beliefs within our worldview through our media, specific cultures, and social systems. It can be beliefs and attitudes about race, religion or spiritual affiliation, political ideology, cultural practices or values, gender-based behaviors, age, socio-economic status, disability, and so on. We also have primitive cognitive processes that play against us in this fight because we are hardwired to categorize our world to identify threats and opportunity for survival. What we are capable of is creating more awareness

DOI: 10.4324/9781003001881-3

around these biases and accepting their existence. By accepting the existence of these biases, one can remove the feelings of shame that prevent progressive dialogue. When a person feels shame for an unconscious bias, the first reaction is to defend oneself because of the perceived threat of social persecution or being labeled.

One of the most cited and groundbreaking works about prejudice is Gordon Allport's *The Nature of Prejudice* (1954). He wrote that categorical thinking is an inevitable process of the human mind. Allport introduced concepts linking acts of prejudice and one's world view, and he postulated that prejudice is primarily a result of a general *motivated cognitive style*. Characteristics of this motivated cognitive style include a need for familiarity, low tolerance for ambiguity, desire and drive for quick and precise answers, strong preference for organization and social order, and fear of not knowing or understanding something. Allport also suggested that people with this rigid type of personality style could not overcome prejudiced thinking or benefit from increased contact and exposure to different groups of people (Allport, 1954). This cognitive style essentially seeks security through pulling personal anecdotal information and reasoning from a mental reservoir to inform oneself of the best course of action. The person using this cognitive style will then perceive themselves to have more control of the outcome. Some criticism for Allport's work comes from his notion that prejudice is a personality type that is permanent rather than a behavior that we are all capable of based in a primitive cognitive process within our brains.

The need for cognitive closure (NFC), a theory proposed by Donna Webster and Arie Kruglanski (1995), explains that a person would rather have an answer, any answer, to something rather than ambiguity or confusion. The level of need for closure is related to the perceived benefits, cost, or both, and the need for closure intensifies as the need for predictability and action arises (Webster & Kruglanski, 1995). The NFC theory has been foundational in psychology for understanding human decision making and judgment. There are two types of tendencies that relate to the action of making judgments. One is *urgency*, which arises from the need to have definitive and quick answers, leaving a person vulnerable to accept any information available that fulfills this need. The second is *permanence*, which is the action of defending and preserving the information acquired despite given information that challenges the ideas. NFC has been linked to racism and sexism, and people who show high-NFC resort to *essentialist categorization* and *authoritarian ideologies* in social environments to achieve closure. These two behaviors are highly linked to determining prejudice and stereotyping. Roets and Van Hiel (2011) summarize what I am attempting to convey about prejudice: "Social categorization allows people to construct and organize knowledge about the social world and to cope with its complexity" (p. 351). The categorization process suggests that these mental filing cabinets provide concrete understanding and definitions that are assigned to entire groups of people. This in turn leads to essentialism, or creating absolutes, which inspires prejudiced and stereotypical thinking (Roets & Van Hiel, 2011).

Let's sum up the motivational and cognitive process that contributes to prejudice. Ambiguity reduces the sense of safety and security due to its lack of predictability. Uncertainty, or a lack of clear rules and boundaries, elicits anxiety. Anxiety, in any context, is an advocate for survival, so it encourages us to analyze threats and opportunities, and then construct and implement a plan for success. In order to increase odds of survival, our brain categorizes everything we experience into a mental filing cabinet so that we know what to avoid, how to react when faced with danger, and seek opportunities that bring rewards. Our mental filing system craves simple absolutes because it feels more efficient. However, it does not keep up with the complexity of our world and doesn't do justice to our unique social experiences. This process, in addition to other social and cultural factors that lead to or encourage essentialist thinking, manifests stereotyping and prejudice.

All social interactions require risk taking, ranging on a spectrum from low-risk to high-risk behaviors. The intensity of these risks is determined by the level of vulnerability that is required. Higher social risks demand more vulnerability, and uncertainty tends to follow acts of vulnerability due to the unpredictability of the recipient's response. Ambiguity about the outcome is at the heart of shared vulnerability in social scenarios.

A high-risk social interaction has high ambiguity and requires higher levels of vulnerability. Some examples of high-risk social interactions are:

Not knowing ideas or values about a person prior to engaging with them.

One that requests higher level of personal disclosure or sharing of intimacy.

Increased probability of a potentially negative response or outcome.

Outcome of a negative interaction has high stakes consequences of person's emotional state or ego.

A low-risk social interaction has less ambiguity and more certainty. Some examples of low-risk social interactions are:

There is a high predictability of the outcome of the social interaction.

One that requires less vulnerability, leaving less room for intense emotional consequences.

Intimate sharing was earned after secure and safe context was established. This could have been achieved with time and familiarity, level of connection of intimacy, or context of relationship (like a therapist or other professional).

As social animals, humans are often motivated by social connection and positive interactions; we all want to be liked and to feel included.

Relatability decreases the level of risk, which is why people tend to gravitate towards those who share similarities. We want to be able to read people quickly so we can decide whether they are a high-risk or low-risk social opportunity. Because of this inherent motivation and the way our brains work, we are not free of prejudice. Social prejudices are created through the intricate cognitive processes that are motivated by deeper needs.

This does not let anyone off the hook for acting on prejudices. Rather, this information is intended to create understanding and empower individuals to identify, challenge, and deconstruct their own prejudices. My intent is to encourage the practice of welcoming new contradictory evidence and information that boosts more expansive and inclusive thinking—not perceiving such information as a threat to avoid or dismiss new information, but one that invites a spectrum of identities and social opportunities. This information also helps clinicians working with marginalized populations form positive connotations of individuals who resist more expansive ideas. Having positive connotations of clients makes them easier to work with and provides mental health professionals material to work within facilitating change.

Let's apply this to gender. I'm sure everyone has heard the phrase "gender is a social construct." This is true. Gender differs from sex. Sex is the biological "meat sack" we are assigned according to our chromosomes. Sex determines primary and secondary sex characteristics and is relevant in topics of biology and medicine. Gender is more about defining social experiences and interactions, and it inspires aspects of personal identity gained from belonging to the social category. It is an over-simplified and rigid box that has origins in reproductive opportunity, role distribution, and social organization. Gender has been divided into two opposing boxes (man or woman) with low opportunity for flexibility—the *gender binary*. Once placed in either category, there is an entire rule book of behavior, expression, and values assigned to an individual; it is taught to children and policed by adults. We do not give ourselves enough credit for how complex and unique our brains and identities are, and because of this lack of expansive thinking, gender diverse populations suffer.

I once believed that this distribution served humans well at one time, giving myself a reason for the formation of the gender binary. This belief was created and reinforced by our culture, media, and education system. But now I know this isn't true if you look at the history of inclusion of multiple genders within indigenous and historical cultures around the world. To identify a few, there are the *hijra* in South Asia, the *muxe* of the Zapotec people in Mexico, the *mahu* of Hawaii, *kathoey* in Thailand, *bakla* in the Philippines, the *fa'afatama* and *fa'afafine* of Samoan people, and the *waria* in Indonesia. Also present in Indonesia are the Buginese people of South Sulawesi who incorporate five genders into their social organization, including a gender transcendent category of *bissu*. Of the Native Americans, the *two-spirit* people were forced into hiding by colonization, and unfortunately this group of people are not the only group to lose such critical aspects of their culture as a result of colonization. Many of these cultures incorporated expansive gender identities into their culture as sacred, spiritual, and shamanic leaders; colonization sought to destroy their existence. So in reality, a binary division of gender did not serve humans any better than expansive inclusion of gender.

Anticipate that internal prejudice will happen. It's a natural cognitive process. Most times it will be an "oh, wow I didn't know that existed" moment that presents a learning opportunity for you and how you perceive the world. The critical practice of seeking expansive wisdom is to accept and deeply consider challenges to your way of thinking that ends with growth. Perspective is reality. Inclusive multi-perceptive taking expands one's reality and truth. Understand that prejudice is at the heart of social categorization, because if we can fit our world into tidy neat boxes we feel more secure and safe. Humans are deluded by the idea that we can predict social experiences by reducing everyone we encounter into narrow stereotypical definitions. Gender is just another cognitive filing process we rely on in our social interactions and relationships. If our brains are not yet evolved past this behavior, then we need to add more boxes to our repertoire.

For cisgender clinicians working with trans clients, the concept of privilege is a crucial dynamic in the therapeutic relationship to be aware of. As a cisgender therapist, I will never be fully capable of understanding the deeply complex and unique issues of navigating our world as trans. Because of this knowledge, I understood early in my professional development that I would always be a student to not only the developing research and ever-changing visibility of information, but a student of my clients. This book is influenced by my personal and professional experiences. My perception will always be impacted by the privilege of being a white, cisgender, and able-bodied woman. Professionals need to expand their education to include a variety of trans narratives and voices. Especially listen to trans black, indigenous, and people of color (BIPOC), whose histories and narratives have been hijacked and erased as they suffer the most violent and oppressive consequences of transphobia. Listen to trans people with disabilities, individuals who suffer chronic abuse and invisibility. My clients have taught me, and continue to teach me, the majority of what I know and understand about the impact of navigating gender actualization in our oppressive society. Their influence is ever present in my professional practice and clinical approaches. It is necessary for clinicians when working with any marginalized population to be aware of the impact of privilege on our perceptions and to learn to be vulnerable and accept challenges. This practice will expand our understanding and world view beyond our own narratives.

Privilege is not the dismissal of person's hardships, trauma, or any additional adversity, it is the presence of an upper hand dealt by sheer luck. I use an activity with my students to teach this concept by splitting them into groups with an assigned dollar amount I give each group. I then provide a sheet consisting of social, medical, and legal accommodations that students must buy with their dollar amount. Essentially, the group members who were given wealth get more accommodations than those assigned with poverty. We cannot choose the systems we are born into, and we naturally get more benefits if we are born into environments with more societal advantages. Discussion of privilege is exactly this, not a criticism to any suffering a person has endured. It seems the most defensiveness I have encountered in discussions about privilege stem from a person feeling dismissed for overcoming some form of adversity in life and diminishing their accomplishment; this could include advancements in financial status, career, education, family and relationships, or personal rewards. I also notice that denial of privilege stems from the deep fear of shame, perse-cution, and being labeled for being a perpetuator of something negative. I can validate this fear since there is a real toxic culture of public shaming plaguing social media, while I also support the practice of returning voices and power to individuals it's been stripped from. Discussion of privilege is not this simple "all or nothing" topic, it is highly complex and based in multiple systems. It's about people who are chronically at a disadvantage because of who they are in a society with a rigid and unwavering value system.

Intersectionality is the multiple "intersecting," or interconnecting, of layers of oppression and disadvantages a person experiences for being a part of more than one marginalized group. This results in strengthening power of the privileged groups who gained their advantages from the sys-temic marginalization and oppression of marginalized groups of people. These groups can include race, ethnicity, disability, sex, gender identity, attraction or sexual orientation, size, age, socio-economic status, mental health or medical hardships, education, and religious or spiritual affili-ation. If a person belongs to more than one group disadvantaged in our society, they are experiencing intersectionality. The important concept when considering intersectionality is that you cannot focus solely on one aspect of a person's experience or identity; rather, understand that the privileges and oppressions a person encounters overlap. For example, a cisgender, white male who is gay has the cultural advantages associated with being cisgender, male, and white, but also faces the disadvantages of being gay in our society. So, when working with trans populations, it's important to consider the entire picture because it will impact the narrative and process of addressing *gender actualization* in treatment.

Gender actualization is the social, expressive, and existential process of becoming one's liberated and authentic self through the context of gender identity. This process only sometimes includes physical or medical interventions, most of the time includes social integration of some kind, and always includes existential and identity for alignment and congruence. *Transition* is also used interchangeably within gender therapy to encom-pass this unique process of integrating one's gender identity into their life. The term transition doesn't do enough justice to the entirety of experiences trans people go through as they pursue wholeness. While writing an article with a colleague, we decided to begin using this term to better describe what's really going on deep within the individual and to use transition to describe the checklist items or logistics within the innerworkings of gender actualization.

Clinicians reading this must recognize the overlap of Maslow's *self-actualization*, or the human need for self-fulfillment by meeting their full potential, ultimately pursuing and becoming their best self (Maslow, 1943). This is the simplified version, as the theory of self-actualization is a subject of philosophical debate due to how it is interpreted. To actualize a critical aspect of oneself is the beginning of a new step towards self-discovery, and for trans populations, this is essentially what happens when the gender identity is actualized or realized. Maslow's ideas about self-actualization were the direct inspiration for gender actualization, which is at the core of affirming gender therapy.

It is critical that gender therapists use affirming and correct language and terminology as it is a crucial trust-building process for the therapeutic relationship. The Sapir–Whorf Hypothesis of Linguistic Relativity postulates that our language influences our world view and how we perceive and think about experiences (Hussein, 2012). This means that when we use a certain set of language, the words and terminology we use will influence how we think, feel, and experience the world. This can be closely linked to my previous deconstruction of prejudice. If someone continues to use a term that is derogatory or unaffirming about a person or group, that language is internalized by the user, and the user of that term will experience individuals of that group as the definition or meaning of the word choices. For example, if someone continues to misgender a transwoman (not using she/her/hers in reference to her), they will foster a transphobic prejudice that she is somehow not a woman. Using correct pronouns for all genders will encourage internalizing expansive perspectives about gender. Applying linguistic relativity to affirming therapy means that if clinicians are mindful and conscious about language, then they will internalize more inclusive and diverse information about the world and their clients.

When training new clinicians, one of the first concepts I emphasize is language because it can make or break a trusting space. When a client feels safe and affirmed by their clinician, it's because they feel seen for who they are authentically. There will be times when a clinician is challenged with using correct names and pronouns. Sometimes a client might change their identified name and pronoun in the middle of treatment as they grow more comfortable, and other times it may be due to contextual preferences the client requests. Individuals newer to the field may fumble at first until the familiarity with expressive incongruence sets in. I ask trainees to purposefully use the client's identified name and pronouns consciously in sessions, while also being careful to not exaggerate or overuse names and pronouns in session. Trainees are also instructed to use the client's identified name and pronouns in documentation as soon as the client has disclosed them to the clinician (usually this done in the initial demographic paperwork). Training the brain to use this language will begin to create easier association even when the gender expression and the gender identity of the client are not stereotypically congruent; this is how I integrate the linguistic relativity theory. After some time in the field, I noticed that I experience someone for their gender identity beyond their presenting expression at any given time. For example, it is common for clients to feel uncomfortable expressing their authentic gender presentation until progress is made towards transition goals. This can create an air of incongruence (between gender expression and gender identity) for newer gender therapists. For myself and my trainees, we have found that once the client's authentic name and pronouns are being used in treatment, it doesn't matter how the client expresses themselves outwardly, we still experience our client as the gender they identify with. This is most likely due to some sort of cognitive process like suggested in the theory of linguistic relativity.

My hope for including the subjects of prejudice, privilege, intersectionality, and linguistic relativity is to bring concreteness and normalcy to cognitive and social processes that impact all people, including gender therapists. Clinicians are not above these experiences and behaviors even though we sometimes like to think we are. These themes will be ever-present and are foundational concepts all gender therapists must be aware of to provide specialized care. If we are asking our clients to deconstruct narratives of internalized shame, transphobia, transmisogyny, additional compounded narratives due to intersectionality, and the thousands of negative messages ingrained from society and family of origin, we need to understand where to even begin. It is the responsibility of gender affirming therapists to learn the skills to assist our clients in understanding that society is the problem, not our clients. Clinicians need to persistently combat the pathological perspective of a normal human identity in sessions.

To conclude this chapter, I am including some tables to review some terminology. I am not including most of the standard 101 terminology as that would quickly descend into its own chapter and that's not the purpose of this book. Instead, I am going to include terms and language I will frequently refer to in this book. Some of it may be familiar to the seasoned clinicians and some of it may not. Language is constantly expanding and evolving as folx of the LGBTQ+ population reclaim and define language that best affirms their experiences. It's not my place to weigh in on those changes, but rather try my best to stay informed, updated, and educated. I'm sure in five years some of these terms will have changed or be under debate. I used to use the asterisk at the end of "trans*" and "LGBTQ*" in an attempt to be inclusive, and that has since been mostly out of practice as it represents "other" instead of being inclusive of a spectrum. Use of "other" is frowned upon in working with marginalized groups because it is experienced as dismissive rather than inclusive. Trans is inherently inclusive enough of the gender diversity umbrella and the "+" for LGBTQ+ is currently used as a more expansive way to include all who identity within the LGBTQ+ population. I'll also add that there are still several folx who continue to use the asterisk when describing themselves or identity, so I am just following the herd the best I can.

Outdated Language

Outdated language includes terminology that is no longer used or acceptable, and it is considered unaffirming to use. Many will notice that I did not include *gender dysphoria* in Table 2.1. I use gender dysphoria for diagnostic or other clinical purposes only. Gender dysphoria is a fancy way to describe someone who is experiencing distress and discomfort related to gender. The existence of this diagnosis helps trans people navigate the medical system to get access to appropriate and necessary care. Until the medical system changes to acknowledge trans care as a medical right rather than a mental health condition, this diagnosis will continue to be needed. I take a firm stance in supporting the informed consent model for trans health care, and this will be touched on in later chapters.

Affirming Language

Affirming language goes beyond the textbook-appropriate words; it requires the clinician to know how and when to mirror client language. Sometimes clients have reclaimed language or identify strongly with language that affirms them, and it's not up to the clinician to define the person's experience by changing their language. There's a fine line in providing education for newly actualized folx and pressuring a perspective on a person. Affirming language normalizes and replaces words that carry stigma and exclusion and is often left purposely somewhat ambiguous to allow for flexibility and inclusion. When in doubt, I will mirror terms my clients use towards them. Many continue to use "pass" and "stealth" or FTM and MTF.

An interesting example is encouraging more ambiguous language about significant others. Ambiguity seems counterintuitive when there is also specificity to affirming language. In some cases, vagueness can decrease the power or focus on gender-specific language to be more inclusive to nonbinary populations. Of course, the best outcome once language evolves would be terminology that embraces all genders, such as using "spouse" or "partner" for significant others. More than once earlier in my career, I was challenged for using these terms because certain clients felt invalidated by my shift to more ambiguous labels. There is a long history for gay, bi, and lesbian individuals of being forced to hide the identity of their romantic partners for their safety. Not using gender-specific terms can be read by these individuals as a microaggression, as it often is in the realms of family and everyday life. There are also trans folx who want gender-specific nouns to affirm their binary gender identity. As a clinician, we are responsible for

Table 2.1 Outdated terminology and suggested replacements

Outdated Terms	Why?	Try Instead
Preference Preferred Lifestyle	Insinuates choice which dismisses the legitimacy of one's identity. Invalidating.	Ask for name and pronoun without "preferred," What are your pronouns? Share personal pronouns when introducing self. I also use "identified" to differentiate from legal/assigned name and pronouns.
Transgendered Transgenders Intersexed	Reduces person to being trans or intersex as sole aspect of who one is.	Trans person, transgender individual, trans folx, intersex person • People who are intersex are not always trans and do not always identify with LGBTQ+.
Sex change Sex Reassignment Surgery (SRS)	Not affirming language	Gender Affirming Surgery (GAS) Gender Confirmation Surgery (GCS)
Opposite or the other sex Both sexes	Reinforces binary ideas of sex. Lacks inclusivity.	Another sex or a different sex
Opposite or the other gender Both genders	Reinforces binary ideas of gender. Lacks inclusivity.	Another gender or a different gender
Pass Stealth	Perpetuates idea that trans people are somehow deceiving the world and suggests hiding something.	Being seen. Some argue "blending" or "assimilating" is acceptable. • Some trans people still use pass and stealth, mirror client language.
Biological or genetic male/female Born male/female	Unaffirming and invalidating. Overly simplified and generic ways to define sex and gender that aren't completely accurate.	Assigned male/female at birth Designated male/female at birth Or use affirming terminology of how a trans person identifies now, as many terms for binary genders, such as transwoman, insinuate the person transitioned from an assigned sex at birth.
FTM (female to male) MTF (male to female)	Overly simplistic and invalidates gender identity. Assigned sex is only necessary for private medical matters and is not relevant information a person has to disclose.	Man, Woman Transman, Transwoman Trans masculine, Trans feminine Transgender woman, Transgender man

Table 2.2 Nonaffirming vs. affirming language

Nonaffirming terms	Affirming language
Breasts	Chest
Vagina	Genitals
Penis	Genitalia
Male/Female Reproductive Organs	Reproductive Organs (without sex identifier)
	Uterus
	Ovaries
	Testes
Beard	Facial Hair
Wig	Hair
Male/Female descriptions of body	Influenced or impacted by testosterone/estrogen
Gender (in binary contexts)	Genders, includes all gender variance

mirroring language of clients to be affirming. See Table 2.2 for affirming and unaffirming language.

Casual Language

Casual language includes more than just shortened words to make things easier to say and write; there are also terms used by the community that are purposefully left vague to be more inclusive and expansive. Sometimes casual language includes words that are only okay to use by individuals who are part of the community. Reclaimed language is the practice of taking back power through words that was once used to oppress a marginalized group. For people who are not trans or of the LGBTQ+ community, reclaimed terms are not for you to use unless you are using them within an educational or appropriate social context such as using term because someone identifies with or of it. Queer is a great example of a reclaimed and casual term. Context is incredibly important for nontrans and non-LGBTQ+ individuals in using this term. Using queer to refer to the LGBTQ+ and trans community as an umbrella term is mostly acceptable to use. It is also acceptable when a person identifies and/or labels themself as a queer identity. It is not acceptable or appropriate to use queer to refer to a person who has not identified themself as a queer identity, with negative or oppressive connotation (unintentional or intentional), or casually/playfully when you are not part of the oppressive group. Below is a list of some widely used and clinically appropriate casual language (even for cis clinicians) (Table 2.3).

To work with disadvantaged populations who require specialized and highly informed care, mental health professionals must first understand and work through their own unconscious biases. Clinicians must first accept

Table 2.3 Casual terms

Casual terms	Meaning
Top Surgery	Surgery to remove chest or augment breasts to affirm gender identity.
Bottom Surgery	Surgery to alter genitalia and/or remove reproductive organs to affirm gender identity.
T	Testosterone
HRT	Hormone Replacement Therapy
Cis	Cisgender, someone who is not trans and gender identity aligns with assignment at birth.
Queer	Reclaimed word with many uses. It can be an umbrella term for the LGBTQ+ community, trans community, nonbinary genders, anyone who doesn't fall into the straight and cis category. It is purposely left ambiguous to be inclusive.
Trans	A very large and diverse spectrum to include all sorts of varying gender identities and expressions. Term encompasses all binary and nonbinary genders that are not exclusively cis.
Folx	A means of addressing a group of people with inclusion to all genders. Often used specifically in contexts where one is purposefully practicing inclusion.
Policing	To enforce or impose rigid and/or oppressive social rules. This can be through persecution. This behavior is practiced by people of the same or different groups. Marginalized groups often struggle with internal policing of one another.

they are not immune to cognitive processes that cause prejudices so that they can successfully dismantle the perpetuation of oppression. Addressing personal experiences of the themes of privilege, intersectionality, prejudice, and unconscious bias is a mandatory ongoing work for gender therapists. By becoming familiar with these truths, and even addressing uncomfortable familiarity with these internal attitudes, therapists can better serve clients and perform their role in helping clients challenge internalized stigma. Making practical changes to language and world view will increase the quality of care marginalized clients will receive.

Reflection Questions for Clinicians

1 How do you feel about the vulnerability that is required to do this work—taking a humbled stance in acknowledging your own prejudices?
2 How can you create more inclusivity in your language, or personal and professional life.
3 What unconscious biases have you noticed or currently hold about trans people?

References

Allport, G. (1954). *The nature of prejudice*. Reading, MA: Addison-Wesley.

Hussein, B. A. (2012). The Sapir-Whorf hypothesis today. *Theories and Practice in Language Studies*, 2(3), 642–646.

Maslow, A. H. (1943). A theory of human motivation. *Psychological Review*, 50(4), 370–396, http://psychclassics.yorku.ca/Maslow/motivation.htm

Roets, A., & Van Hiel, A. (2011). Allport's prejudiced personality today: need for closure as the motivated cognitive basis of prejudice. *Current Directions in Psychological Science*, 20(6), 349–354. Retrieved from www.jstor.org/stable/23213072

Webster, D. & Kruglanski, A. (1995). Individual differences in need for cognitive closure. *Journal of Personality and Social Psychology*, 67, 1049–1062. doi: 10.1037/0022-3514.67.6.1049

3 Affirmative Therapy

Expanding Beyond the Gender Binary

Creating a more expansive perspective of gender asks the clinician to challenge and deconstruct stereotypical societal norms about binary gender that are ingrained from birth. Doing so gives an individual an immense amount of room for creativity of expression of self. Gender studies is a great start for this process. Gender is a social construct, and because it is a social construct, our brains have a categorization process for it. Humans love security, and black and white (or binary) thinking provides that security by giving a mental framework that can predict and perceive the world around us with concrete and tangible rules. The twist is that we create these rules and our brain follows suit by creating mental boxes to organize and label the world around us. To best challenge this process, we need to change the socially constructed "rules" to be more fluid in nature by expanding our boxes. We need to increase the quantity and capacity of them.

The gender binary is the fixed and rigid categorization of gender into two opposing groups defined by masculinity and femininity. When defining gender, people have heavily relied on sex, or the primary and secondary sex characteristics a person is assigned at birth. Beyond infants, children and teens are heavily policed by peers and adults to conform to inflexible social expectations assigned to them based on assigned sex. These rules are inspired by socially constructed ideals of femininity and masculinity. Masculinity is assigned to men and femininity is assigned to women, and if either strays from their assigned seat there will be consequences depending on the nature of the offense. Masculine and feminine are two sides of the same coin, recognized as a complimentary experience in spiritual practices and ancient and sacred lore. They are meant to be symbiotic within one person, but this concept has been hijacked to romanticize cis and straight narratives; completion can only occur when a man and a woman come together, not when these forces are joined within a single person. Essentially, the gender binary includes two boxes: man and woman. Affirming gender practices continues to recognize these two classifications, while expanding them a bit to include cisgender and transgender men and women. Expanding upon the gender binary, there is now a new system of

DOI: 10.4324/9781003001881-4

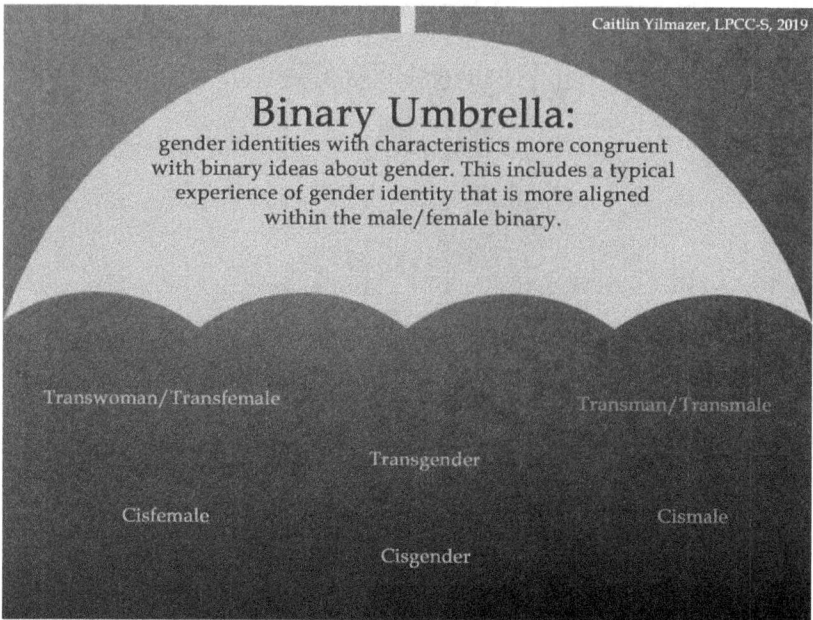

Figure 3.1 Binary genders umbrella.

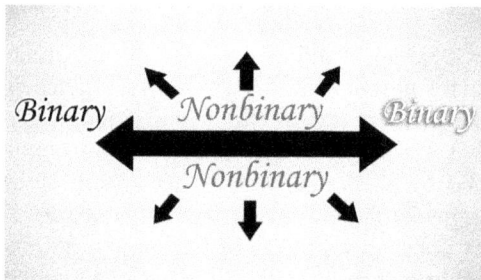

Figure 3.2 Binary and nonbinary spectrum. When referring to gender specifically, the concept of nonbinary can go beyond the spectrum.

gender classification that encourages more expansive ideas about gender: binary and nonbinary genders (see Figures 3.1 and 3.2).

Nonbinary and Binary Spectrums

Transgender and *cisgender* are binary terms. In Latin, "cis-" is a prefix meaning "the same side of" or "on this side," supporting its definition of a person whose gender identity aligns with their assigned sex at birth. The

Latin prefix "trans-" means across or to cross over, which can describe a transgender person who transitions because of a lack of alignment in gender identity and assigned body at birth. What might get a little confusing is "trans-" can also mean "beyond" or "transcendent," which compliments nonbinary genders. *Transgender* is still a binary gender term and *trans* is more expansive and inclusive, including both binary and nonbinary populations. I will be using these terms purposefully throughout this book, understanding the difference is important.

Nonbinary gender includes gender nonconforming identities that do not fit or go beyond society's binary expectations and ideas about gender. The nonbinary category includes another set of possibilities such as multiple genders, no gender, neutral genders, fluid genders, partial genders, transcendent genders, culturally and spiritually specific genders, and gender nonconformity (see Figure 3.3). Essentially the nonbinary realm has fewer rules by nature than the other genders, but that means these folx tend to experience significant external policing and sometimes they are policed even within the LGBTQ+ community. This results in a severe lack of social accommodation, higher incidents of identity dismissal, and invisibility. Culturally and spiritually specific genders are exampled in Chapter 1, such as two-spirit in Native American culture. When addressing culturally specific genders, it's important to understand that individuals who are not of that culture cannot really define or accurately conceptualize that gender identity because they do not have the appropriate lens. For example, I cannot fully describe the two-spirit gender since I am not of a culture that includes it, even my language would be limited and coming from a person whose culture still heavily enforces rigid binary ideas about gender. Some people tend to describe two-spirit peoples as transgender but this is not accurate because it's oversimplified.

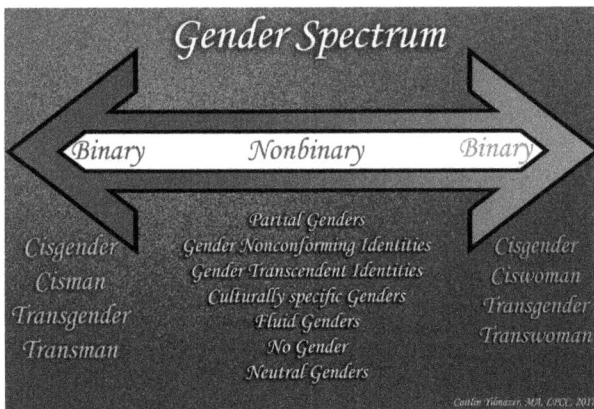

Figure 3.3 Binary and nonbinary gender spectrums.

Intersex is an umbrella term used to describe individuals who were born with primary and/or secondary characteristics that are not congruent with binary expectations of sex. The notion of dimorphic, or two forms, of sex is incorrect. This is yet another example of the complex and diverse human experience. According to the Intersex Society of North America (ISNA):

> If you ask experts at medical centers how often a child is born so noticeably atypical in terms of genitalia that a specialist in sex differentiation is called in, the number comes out to about 1 in 1500 to 1 in 2000 births. But a lot more people than that are born with subtler forms of sex anatomy variations, some of which won't show up until later in life.

Because of our dimorphic notions about sex, intersex individuals have suffered greatly. Decisions have been made by parents and medical professionals to perform non-medically necessary surgeries to alter sex characteristics of infants and children, resulting in severe consequences. Surgical intervention poses several problems including the permanency of the alterations, impact to sexual functioning, trauma, identity issues, and is a violation of the person's autonomy. When working with individuals who are intersex, do not assume they identify as trans. The spectrum of intersex conditions is quite large and there are many folx who do not identify as trans or experience concerns about gender identity. There have also been cases of an intersex person identifying as trans because they were deprived of their autonomy because of early surgical intervention, forcing a transition and gender actualization process. *Amalgagender* is a gender identity where the person has integrated intersex experience and gender identity.

Another important concept to understand is that all gender identities allow fluidity; it doesn't matter if it is a nonbinary or binary gender identity. Just as society is coming to embrace the fluidity of human sexuality, gender identity is no different. Binary and nonbinary gender identities have room for some flexibility in how they experience their gender identity. Binary gender identities have room for fluid experiences, and these individuals often experience policing that ignites doubt and stress. Inexperienced therapists might see this fluidity and unintentionally inspire doubt by questioning the legitimacy of the client's gender identity. This type of policing fosters the negative "am I trans enough" narrative that clients grapple with as they actualize their gender. We can all agree that humans are deeply complex creatures, so it's perfectly normal for complexity to be present in our identities and personalities. We are all unique, walking contradictions of our categorization behaviors.

Affirmative Therapy

The affirming clinician understands that gender identity is an inherent aspect of a person that cannot be changed. Affirming therapists have an unconditional positive regard for their client's identity. Finally, the affirming professional has concrete understanding that gender is fluid and unique in all individuals, including both binary and nonbinary folx. Clinicians adopting this orientation affirm and support clients for how they identify and feel authentically to provide the space to explore and process their sense of self. When clients in the early phases of gender actualization come to treatment, they are incredibly vulnerable to the influence of their clinician. In affirmative therapy, the clinician is required to be very aware of society's negative impact on their clients to help facilitate a de-programing and deconstruction of negative internalized messages. Some professionals argue that dysphoria only exists because of society, while others challenge the very distinct physical sensation of incongruence would continue to persist even in a diverse gender society. Regardless, in the world we interact with now, the current culture instills toxic messages of transphobia and transmisogyny in gender diverse folx.

Adopting the affirmative orientation is more than implementing "LGBTQ+-friendly" values, it's taking the time to acquire specialty. There's a difference in a trauma-informed clinician and a trauma certification. It requires intensive personal, educational, and clinical work and practice to acquire affirmative therapy specialization. Below are some expectations of a practicing affirming clinician.

The gender affirming therapist has expertise in the construction and deconstruction of gender.

For cisgender therapists, a helpful starting point is learning how to deconstruct the cis-normative expectations about men and women. Once this glass-shattering moment happens, that rush of reality reveals that the structures surrounding gender assignment are quite flawed and oppressive to all involved. No one really wins. Toxic masculinity is a deeply disturbing and harmful form of masculinity rooted in a traditional perspective of what men should be. It often results in emotional repression, lack of intimate connection and close friendships, aggressive or domineering performance, violent policing, enforcing or perpetuating misogyny, seeking power to obtain value, pursuit of dominance through oppressive actions and beliefs against minorities and women, and beliefs that financial contribution is their primary purpose and value. Toxic masculinity isn't just damaging to society, it's extremely harmful to boys and men. Recognizing this real problem, the American Psychological Association released a publication of guidelines in 2018 for professionals to implement in their practice to combat the repercussions of toxic masculinity, though it's more gently referred to as "traditional" and "dominant" masculinity in the document. The damaging impact of toxic masculinity includes high rates of substance abuse, violence, incarceration, mortality, receiving harsher punishments, mental health issues, suicide rates, physical health issues, relationship and family problems, academic problems, dropouts, and barriers in seeking help

(American Psychological Association, 2018). While it is important to recognize the privilege of men, this barely scratches the surface of intersecting influences on how men perform their masculinity.

When a clinician can deconstruct the binary cisgender categories, their understanding of the complex issues of transgender people will increase. For binary transgender people, not only is the person dealing with internalized oppressive gender constructs that they were assigned from birth, they are also trying to navigate the territory of the gender with which they identify. To effectively work with these clients, the specialized affirming clinician needs to understand the social construct of gender like the back of their hand in order to help clients effectively sort through the onslaught of gender experiences from the past, present, and future. An affirming gender therapist will sort through the impact of gender experiences for the entire course of treatment, and the way it appears will constantly be changing.

Finally, after thoroughly understanding binary genders, the clinician can then grasp the complexity of nonbinary genders. Remember, this realm includes the possibility of multiple genders, no gender, neutral genders, fluid genders, partial genders, transcendent genders, culturally and spiritually specific genders, and gender nonconformity. After learning how to deconstruct the actual construct of gender, the affirming gender therapist should be able to simply understand the variety of gender experiences with which one can identify. Nonbinary clients have unique oppressions that are rooted in society's binary division of gender accommodations. There is a complete lack of visibility for nonbinary persons in day-to-day society. This will be more specifically expanded upon in future chapters.

There are several qualifications expected of an affirming gender therapist. The role of a gender-specialized clinician is not to legitimize or label a person as trans. Rather it is to hold a supportive and affirming space so the client can explore and recognize their own identity. Sometimes clinicians can feel pressured to confirm a person's gender identity, but mental health professionals are not psychic nor do they have the means to peek inside the human brain and pinpoint the gender a person experiences. For a clinician to market themselves as a gender therapist, they are responsible for meeting the special qualifications that set them apart from other professionals in the area. This is why the "LGBTQ+ friendly" and ally therapists can cause problems for a client's access to the care they need; this type of marketing can be misleading for folx who are looking for a gender therapist. Allied counselors are great, which means more safe places and support for the LGBTQ+ community; however, they fall short of specific knowledge and skills needed for actual gender therapy. The gender affirming therapist:

- Understands similarities and co-occurring lifespan developmental phases and transition.
- Has knowledge of the process of administrative aspects of transition (legal, documentation, name changes, etc.).

- Is informed about the medical aspects of transition, including effects of HRT and current procedures and options for GAS.
- Recognizes that working with trans populations is working with a high-risk population.
- Knows how one's systems, including culture and a person's family of origin experience, impact how gender identity is conceptualized by the individual.
- Understands how gender and sexuality are different and yet interact with one another.
- Is connected with local community resources and has compiled comprehensive resources for clients that trans folx clinician may interact with.
- Approaches their work with humility and vulnerability, as learning and growth is expected to be ongoing. Working with marginalized populations requires the ability to accept being challenged.

Additionally, gender therapists are expected of the following:

The gender affirming therapist has a strong understanding of the impact of marginalization, privilege, intersectionality, and oppression on our clients.

Expanding upon the information presented in Chapter 1, an experienced affirming clinician realizes the unique impact of the client's systems on their gender actualization process. The therapist then needs to aid clients in challenging and sorting through their complex intersecting experiences to better access and strengthen the authentic self. The trans experience is not one simplistic universal narrative by any means, it's highly impacted by the person's ecological systems. Urie Bronfenbrenner (1979) pioneered the theory of ecological systems, a perspective that suggests a child's development is impacted by their relationship with several systems within the child's environment. These systems include: the *microsystem, mesosystem, exosystem, macrosystem*, and *chronosystem*.

The *microsystem* contains the direct contact structures including family, school, childcare environment, and neighborhood. This layer has the greatest impact on a child and is bi-directional in its influence. This means that both the child's beliefs and behavior are influenced by the relationships and people within these structures, and the child also has influence over the people and relationships within this system. The *mesosystem* is the connection or intersection between the structures within the microsystem, such as church and family or teacher and parent. The *exosystem* is the layer of influence from a system that does not directly impact the child, but rather interacts with another structure in the microsystem. This might be a parent's interaction with their workplace that indirectly influences the child. Community resources are also at this level. The *macrosystem* is the most external system of the child and includes the culture the child is assigned. This includes socioeconomic status, ethnicity, and shared cultural values, laws, and identity. The macrosystem has the ability to expand and change with time and can trickle down and influence other intersecting layers within a child's systems. The *chronosystem* is the transitional events that occur over time that impact the systems. An example could be a progressive societal change that offers more opportunities to a marginalized group. Another example is a divorce or death that causes significant adjustment and change to a person's system (Berk, 2000).

A child is assigned to their systems, meaning we cannot control the circumstances of birth. People are born into a variety of contexts, cultures, communities, and families that impact their world view. Now add the layer of the conceptualization and implementation of gender, and you begin to understand how uniquely complex a person's relationship with their gender identity is. It is the responsibility of the gender affirming clinician to have a deep understanding of this complexity and help the client unravel and challenge all of the damaging internalized messages that are not serving their self-actualizing process.

> *The gender affirming therapist seeks ongoing and up to date information, research, training, community and resource connection, and additional immersion in the information of LGBTQ+ issues.*

Mental health professionals are not offered a lot of specialized education during their programs. These graduate students are expected to seek this information out themselves either during the program for projects of their choice, their internship experience, or post-graduation. Unfortunately, there is a somewhat problematic message which students are given at graduation about working with future clients, which is often reinforced by workplaces and contributes to burnout. The message is that if a clinician doesn't feel competent or seasoned to work with a certain issue a client presents, they are trained well enough to figure it out. Essentially, if you don't feel competent then you need to get competent. In some contexts, this message is completely true and clinicians *should* get competent to help specialized and unique issues that come through the door. But this message also perpetuates a false confidence that clinicians can work with anything and should continue to work with clients instead of referring when it's appropriate. Would you go to your primary care doctor to evaluate and treat a neurological medical problem or a neurologist? Mental health professionals are busy, we don't have time to get specialized or competent in several different therapies because of one new client challenges us. So, the go-to action is to consult with a peer, read a few articles, or attend a training. This just isn't enough for many clients who present a need for specialized care.

While the numbers are steadily increasing, there is a clear lack of trans clinicians. The lack of voices is deafening. This means that the trans perspective in clinical work is also sorely missing from the discourse in gender therapy. That's not to say there are not trans clinicians working to develop this field, there are many intricate levels to oppression that is blocking trans folx from clinical spaces or from the academia. Just like other marginalized groups, trans folx do not receive the same support systematically to excel beyond certain spaces.

To be an effective and experienced affirming gender therapist, it takes more than a training or two. The clinician should continue to consult with a supervisor or peers with experience, continue to read the latest research about the needs of the population, attend any training that would help increase expertise, read books, connect and maintain connections to resources within the community, and try to be involved somehow with the community whether it's advocacy or participating or lurking in online forums. Visibility and language are constantly changing and expanding and the LGBTQ+ community are the leaders and voices of this process.

> *The gender affirming therapist has the ability to maintain a secure sense of self while accepting challenges. They engage in the consistent practice of self-reflection and identification of their own privileges and unconscious biases that influence clients and our world.*

Mindfulness about the presence of one's own privilege in therapeutic settings is a necessary practice for all clinicians in order to be truly effective and person-centered. Working with gender populations, it can be a common experience for a clinician who is cis to experience cisgender guilt. This idea of guilt can expand to other clinical contexts including, but not exclusive to, sexuality, race, ethnicity, culture, socioeconomic status, disability, and mental health history. Privilege guilt typically stems from a guilt of not earning the privileges gained by being an advantaged person. Triggers for this guilt happen when there is information or a confrontation that challenges the privileged person's contribution to perpetuating oppressive experiences of disadvantaged people. When this happens, the person of privilege will sometimes have reactive behavior, in response to the guilt or fear of persecution, which is usually defensive in nature. Gender affirming therapists need to be able to consciously reflect when they are feeling challenged by information that elicits this form of guilt. This interaction will even happen to the most seasoned and experienced therapists.

> *The gender affirming therapist will avoid gatekeeping behaviors as much as possible.*

Because clinicians have been placed strategically between trans folx and access to necessary medical care, we have been forced into the role of gatekeepers. The fact that clients are required to come to us to be deemed mentally and emotionally competent to make decisions about their own bodies and medical care makes us gatekeepers even when we don't want to be. Clinicians are also responsible for our professional processes because we have obligations and duties to our licenses, our work sites, and all the other fun organizations working behind the scenes who assign even more intense rules to our procedures. Because of this, therapists need to be extra careful about their approaches to trans clients. Many of our clients are coming to our office with lack of trust because the very nature of the therapeutic relationship has gatekeeping.

> *The gender affirming professional works to internalize an expansive perspective of gender.*

Lastly, gender therapists need to work on their internalized beliefs, values, and ideas about gender on a personal level. Mental health professionals are not free of the influence of their own values in their work. Because we are human, our values are constantly present in our daily lives. We also need to be aware that we are not superhuman and expect complete enlightenment so that we are free from all of our limiting beliefs. Gender therapists must work on expanding their own perceptions of gender by reflecting on and challenging the existing cis-normative beliefs and opening their mind's spectrum.

Gender is an enigma. It's both highly important and pointless at the same time. While gender is a construct that has the potential to impose highly rigid rules and performance, it is also a deep reservoir of inspiration and creativity for an individual's self-expression. Because our world heavily relies on gender for social interactions, marketing and consumerism, and overall social division and accommodation, embracing our gender identities and having the freedom to express what they mean to us is vital to our wellbeing. How we outwardly express ourselves is a social interaction in itself; it's how we advertise ourselves to others. Our fashion choices, hair styles, tattoos, jewelry, clothing choices, footwear, makeup, and all the other costuming we utilize send messages to our communities about our values and hint at other social categories we belong to. When we subscribe to our gender identity, the message of the gender binary encourages our creativity to be limited to the norms associated with that gender. In reality, if we were to relax, or even eliminate, the strict rules of self-expression and gender, there would only be more creativity available to us to express ourselves freely with less stigma. When a gender therapist can embrace this expansive perspective of gender, see the co-occurring importance and unimportance of its construct, and experience unconditional positive regard for how a person identifies, they can effectively help clients find land among the vast ambiguous sea that is human identity.

Reflection Questions for Clinicians

1   Do you feel like you meet the criteria of what it takes to be an affirming therapist? What areas need development and growth?
2   Identify areas of growth to take a more expansive perspective of gender.

3   When were you first introduced to the concept of intersex conditions? How does this impact your practice or understanding of the dynamic between gender and sex?

References

American Psychological Association, Boys and Men Guidelines Group. (2018). *APA guidelines for psychological practice with boys and men.* Retrieved from: www.apa.org/about/policy/psychological-practice-boys-men-guidelines.pdf

Berk, L. E. (2000). *Child development* (5th ed.). Boston: Allyn and Bacon, 23–38.

Bronfenbrenner, U. (1979). *The ecology of human development: experiments by nature and design.* Cambridge, MA: Harvard University Press.

4 Unique Challenges to Consider

Gender therapists should adopt a lens that adapts to a wide array of ways gender identity is experienced and impacts daily life. Trans populations are considered high risk in a stand-alone state, and when adding intersectional experience, the risk and complexities increase. This impact touches mental health, social accommodations, reproductive opportunities, and culture. By understanding how encompassing gender actualization is for our clients, within every facet of living, we can best support them as they try and fathom what their direction looks like. This chapter outlines some of the unique considerations to think about when working with intersectional experiences that can influence the gender actualization process.

Risk Factors

There is a flooding of new information every year regarding the risk factors for gender diverse populations, adults and youth. The studies, assessments, and demographics collected have a common theme: our current cultural structure is providing an enormous disservice to the trans community. While there are many aspects of our culture evolving and changing to accommodate gender diversity, there is still a long way to go and the longer we are complacent, the longer the trans community suffers. This is the same for all marginalized populations. There is an overwhelming amount of information supporting the following risk factors associated with trans populations, including increased risk for: family rejection (which is also an indicator of the risk level), substance abuse, self-harm, depression, anxiety, suicide attempts and death, physical and sexual assault, abuse, death by homicide, hate crimes, work and housing discrimination, barriers to medical and mental health, poor physical health, risky sexual behaviors, and everything under the sun that occurs as a result of oppressive cultural stigmas and practices. The marginalization and discrimination is multi-faceted; it plagues trans persons occupationally, medically, academically, socially, and legally. The risks expand when talking about gender diverse youth, which is a very vulnerable population.

Gender doesn't define an entire person, but it does provide context for an aspect of a person's identity. While society is starting to expand

DOI: 10.4324/9781003001881-5

gender categories, there are still categories. Until the need for organized structure in our world ends, humans will continue to create and perpetuate categories to make sense of the complexity of our world. And because of this, gender will continue to be an important part of social interactions, and thus an important feature of our identities because we are innately social animals. This is not intended to promote exclusivity, rather to pressure more inclusivity of the spectrum of genders so people can have the space to authentically actualize themselves and their gender identity. When this change occurs, the risk factors associated with the trans population can begin to decrease as the wounds of this community, imposed by transphobic structures and interactions, can begin to heal.

Understanding the disparities between our cisgender and transgender clients is critical in providing affirming treatment for supporting gender diversity. The foundation of gender affirming care is the deconstruction of internalized stigma society imposed upon the trans person by constructs riddled with prejudices. One study by Perez-Brumer, Hatzenbuehler, Oldenburg, and Bockting (2015) suggests that the internalization of transphobia is a primary indicator of risk for suicidality. This study assessed internalized stigma among trans individuals and found that the lifetime suicide attempts were higher among those with higher levels of internalized stigma, and lower among those with lower scores. This study also highlights the stigmas associated with intersectionality and how it impacts suicidality and risk level. Baker (2019) reports data show that trans individuals suffer in significantly disproportionate rates than cis people in mental and physical health. This study also compared insurance coverage between trans and cis people, which is less for trans folx. Overall, this study concluded that trans individuals show a significantly higher rate of poor health and severe mental distress.

Understanding intersectionality of multiple marginalized experiences, and how it informs the trans experience of our clients, is critical. For example, gender norms and expectations of black men and women are different than those of white men and women. The same idea expands to all racial diversity, as each carries its own unique culture of gender. Because of this, the gender actualization process and trans experience will be vastly different. In a study by White et al. (2020), black transgender men were interviewed to gather information about their experiences and perceptions. There were six themes identified and evaluated by researchers in which participants reported impact in racial and gender identity: (a) developing an empowered view of self, (b) navigating double consciousness, (c) having a target on your back, (d) strategies of resilience, (e) culture of silence, and (f) finding quality care. Participants reported that shade of their skin, specifically lighter skin, was more advantageous. Another interesting pattern in these interviews is that participants identified themselves as black first, followed by gender. This supports that race has a significant impact on one's gender identity and actualization process. This study also added that the participants gained a better understanding of their racial identity after coming out as trans. It's important for clinicians working with BIPOC communities to understand the intersectionality between race, culture, and gender. If these subjects cannot integrate in the clinical work, then it will negatively impact the delicate gender actualization process of our clients.

According to a survey in 2011 from National Center for Transgender Equality and National Gay and Lesbian Task Force, the level of discrimination and oppression for black trans people was especially devastating of the populations examined. This population faired the worse in almost every risk factor researched. Some of these factors that exhibited a striking bias in risks for black trans folx included higher rates of poverty, low income, suicide attempts, job loss and bias, harassment and bullying in school, and physical and sexual assault. This survey also highlighted that trans indigenous and people of color were disproportionately at higher odds to experience discrimination economically, in housing and homelessness, public accommodation, and abuse by police and by police prison systems. BIPOC trans people are also more likely to experience barriers to documentation changes, appropriate healthcare (for they have poorer health outcomes), and family rejection. Overall, trans BIPOC experience significantly more oppression and discrimination from society in addition to family and social rejection (Grant et al., 2011).

Family rejection is one of the deepest wounds and trauma that is processed in therapy sessions by members of the LGBTQ+ community. This rejection is a primary indicator for the risk factors I have mentioned above, as family is supposed to be a source of affirmation and nurturing for a developing person. Family is depended on as the critical source of support for an LGBTQ+ person navigating a society that doesn't provide it. In addition to traumas related to violence, family rejection, and assault, trans individuals also experience vicarious and shared trauma of their communities and identity trauma imposed upon them through imposed dysphoria and internalized transphobia in all its forms. Much of white culture has more encouragement for individualism which makes boundary setting easier. While the construct of individualism is problematic in many other aspects, boundary setting can be a useful way to decrease exposure to negative influences when one is actualizing their gender. Nonwhite individuals do not always have the ability to set specific boundaries due to cultural differences, and counselors need to be acutely aware of this. White clinicians can't just easily expect our clients to be able to set boundaries to help cope with negative influences of family rejection. Not only do cultural dynamics influence this, but one's personal systems. Marginalized groups experience such systemic oppression that families stick together for a multitude of reasons.

Folx with disabilities deal with societal erasure and imposed labeling daily. Our culture tends to reduce individuals living with disabilities to that single experience, which is incredibly isolating and limiting. Disability is a natural and common aspect of the human experience and can be a permanent or temporary experience at any stage of life. Providers of this population do best when this message is normalized because it impacts the gender actualization process in many ways. There are significant fears for many being denied access to medical intervention because the medical field still has significant progress to be made to be both gender expansive and progressively supportive for individuals living with disabilities. Certain interventions like HRT or affirming surgeries can interact with particular medical needs and conditions, and modern medicine is sorely lacking in competency in how to adjust interventions to affirm trans patients. Individuals living with disability also deal with being passively deemed as genderless through societal stigmas. Clients with disabilities tend to experience higher rates of gatekeeping because inexperienced clinicians are uncomfortable with some co-occurring diagnoses. Gender affirming therapists recognize that disabilities do not define a person. They are co-occurring with all the other complexities that make up the client's identity. Clinicians should increase comfort levels through understanding gender and disability are two separate experiences within a person. And while these are two individual parts, they are also impacting the individual's understanding of self mutually and intertwined too. Providers should understand the intricate oppressive constructs plaguing this population on a daily basis, including how the medical systems that are supposed to help often coerce and pressure these individuals to seek and idea of conformity in order to receive needed care or resources. Gatekeeping is an all too familiar experience in all facets of daily life.

Age and Stage of Life

An important concept to consider is expanding the idea of culture influencing the perception of gender to age and stage of life. For example, there is an entire group of people, multiple generations worth of people, who did not experience a nonbinary revolution. Being introduced to nonbinary options is critical in challenging personally imposed rigid gender expectations. By expanding gender from a binary spectrum, nonbinary folx have been crucial in liberating gender expansiveness. There are stark differences in attitudes about gender when working with clients of advancing age compared to young adults and teens. While there are most definitely exceptions, from my personal clinical experience I've noticed gender therapy clients of advancing age tend to hold more rigid and fixed ideas about gender. I have not worked with many people who identify as nonbinary who are of advancing age. This means when I work with older clients, I commonly see binary identified transgender individuals who have high expectations for expressive and social transition. There is a delicate manner to approach both affirming the client for their self-actualizing needs (which may be rigid transition goals to achieve expectations surrounding gender expression) and introducing healthier concepts surrounding gender to encourage flexibility. Having fixed and stubborn ideas about gender translates to higher intensity of gender dysphoria symptoms because it leaves more room for perceived failure, and this perceived failure then opens a dam of flooding cognitive distortions and negative self-talk. Younger generations have less pressure to subscribe to unyielding gender norms (they certainly are not free of it though), which has generationally increased comfort with natural fluidity of gender. Both cis and trans folx are embracing more flexibility with gender as time passes.

When addressing inflexible standards surrounding gender, make sure to check-in with yourself to ensure you are first and foremost affirming the client's gender identity. Next, there are affirming ways to challenge gender. First, ongoing psychoeducation is an important and effective way to introduce new ideas. This can be done through talk therapy, worksheets, documentaries, and reading assignments—even assigning journaling reflection prompts. Consider your therapeutic orientation and adjusting learned interventions to encourage exploration of gender. For example, exploring family of origin and history of gender expectations can help with gentle dismantling of adopted oppressive gender attitudes. Standard talk therapy strategies such as strategic challenges, reflexive questioning, and anchoring, and adjusting interventions facilitate to identify how these distortions surrounding gender negatively impact self-perceptions. Do not invest in changing the client's mind because sometimes lived experience is needed first before doing this work. Lived experience sometimes must come first before the client is able to start self-actualizing work.

Trauma and Self-Harm

Trauma is a wound that is inflicted by an event that exceeds one's standard day-to-day distress tolerance threshold. Many describe it as a rug being pulled out from underneath them, or it may feel like free falling into a chaotic abyss without anything to grasp or hold onto. Even though gender diverse individuals do indeed experience significant physical traumas, I want to first touch on psychological or emotional trauma. Traumatic events can happen at any given moment or could be an ongoing persisting event. Trauma can occur after injury, illness, accident, assault, death, loss, abuse, birth, vicariously experiencing a distressing event through story or witness, and any other expected or unexpected terrible event. Traumatic experiences and responses fall on their own respective spectrums and are unique to every individual. Therapists working with trans people are expected to be trauma-informed in their approaches with this population. The trans community has disproportionately high rates of trauma, and reports of trauma, posttraumatic stress disorder (PTSD), and dissociative symptoms are high among trans individuals (Chang, Singh, & dickey, 2018). Not only is the trans population highly vulnerable to trauma because of the associated risk factors associated with the intersecting marginalization statuses, but these folx also endure trauma that is unique specifically to trans experiences.

Clinical Example

James was ready to obtain a letter of support for top surgery. He had been coming to appointments for almost a year and expressed he was ready to take this step. James admitted he was afraid of potential gatekeeping and I reassured him that I had yet to encounter a client reporting a negative experience from this surgeon. James then disclosed he was not worried about the affirming stance of the surgeon, rather he was afraid the surgeon would have concerns about the scars that would be exposed during the surgical evaluation. He went on to explain to me that during puberty he felt so betrayed and disgusted by the betrayal of his body that he began self-harming behaviors (cutting) on his chest. James shared that as his chest continued to grow, the more distraught he would become by the day and he is now only starting to feel connected and love for his body again by pursuing physical alignment in his transition. He was concerned that the surgeon would assign more hoops for him to jump through relating to mental health because he has been used to this type of diversion behavior from other gatekeepers along his journey. Ultimately, the surgeon did not become a gatekeeper and provided him the affirming medical intervention he needed. James' experience with puberty was a physically traumatizing event, his story being a unique one to trans folx.

There is consensus among the affirming mental health and medical communities that going through puberty as the wrong sex is traumatizing. It's not uncommon to have clients with multiple coping methods for this bodily betrayal; I've heard several reports of non-suicidal self-harming, such as cutting, pulling hair, scratching, biting, or burning. Many people can relate to an experience when we have felt out of control of our bodies or that our bodies were failing us. Now multiply the intensity of this experience within the context of the existential impact of self-identity. If our bodies do not align with our identity, how can we feel connected or one with them? For many trans folx, the experience of puberty as the wrong sex is deeply traumatizing to the sense of self that it diminishes the investment in life. If you can't be authentically yourself, what's the point of living? This is why trans populations are considered high-risk populations in mental health. Trans individuals do not get the privilege of having their gender identities affirmed so that they can have a concrete sense of themselves secured to build upon. As a result of this bodily trauma, there is risk of individuals developing eating disorders and chronic self-harming behaviors.

In addition to high risk of trauma, trans individuals have a high risk of eating disorders. Studies such as the one by Diemer, Grant, Munn-Chernoff, Patterson, and Duncan (2015) are showing evidence that trans people are experiencing disproportionately higher rates of eating disorders than cis people. In another publication, data concluded high risk of disordered eating among trans youth, and the higher incidence was associated with increased exposure to stigma and discrimination. Protective factors included higher connectivity to family and caring social support (Watson, Veale, & Saewyc, 2016). Gender actualization involves readdressing the relationship between the actualizing individual and their body. The relationship with the body is not only mending the traumatic bodily rejection, it also entails challenging internalized transphobia, transmisogyny, romanticized cis-normative ideas of binary gender expectations. These internalized messages are stored in souls of our clients and can traumatize the body, causing an array of ways individuals cope ranging from harming the body to completely checking out from the body.

Dissociation is a symptom most commonly associated with trauma, while it also exists in many other contexts to aid in adaptive coping; essentially, it's not exclusive to folx with PTSD diagnoses. Dissociation has a spectrum of its own, ranging from common day-to-day behaviors to severe psychological symptoms and diagnoses. In its most common form, dissociation can be "spacing out" or daydreaming that can happen when we are bored, tired, driving, exercising, contemplation while performing duties of the day, or other activities that remove our focus from the primary task at hand. On the other end of the spectrum, severe dissociation can impact memory and detachment from self and body. While there is a higher risk for trans people to have PTSD and trauma, trans folx who have not experienced a more stereotypically obvious traumatic event can definitely experience trauma-like responses. One of the most common examples of this is the dissociative-esque symptoms trans people can adopt to cope with the trauma of body rejection endured in puberty. It is common when talking with clients to hear about a lack of connection with their body; typically this begins as soon as the personal experience with body betrayal began. Mindfulness that incorporates presence with body (though helpful and probably awesome for future treatment) may not be appropriate for individuals early in their actualization process. This intervention should be strongly considered prior to initiating if the individual has comorbid PTSD or severe dissociative symptoms that need other specialized care. Connecting with one's body as a trans person is a very sacred and vulnerable act and should be visited once the person is ready. If a clinician is not trauma informed, specifically regarding trauma in trans populations, there is a high risk for retraumatization and regression.

Resilience

When addressing the mental health needs of any individual, the instinctual reaction is to explore and assess a problem, to pinpoint the symptoms that are causing distress and impairment to the functioning of our clients. This is because of the lingering influence of pathological approaches to mental health that is rooted deep into our profession's history. It is critical to remember that after all this talk of trauma and struggles, trans folx are incredibly and courageously resilient. Resilience is often described as one's strength, or the ability to rebound or recover from adversity and hardship. One of the most important notions to understand about gender diverse populations is the innate resilience imposed upon these individuals by simply existing in a structured culture that favors binary cisnormativity and heteronormativity; this doesn't even scratch the surface of all the privileges gained by intersectional identities and happenstances. As mental health professionals, we are often assessing the internal coping strategies, both effective and ineffective, that have dutifully served our clients in their quest for survival and self-actualization. External support is an important piece to recognize for this population as well due to the impact family, social support, access to affirming resources, and community support have on positive mental health outcomes. Context has everything to do with resilience—intersecting oppressions, culture, family background, personality, experience with adversity, privilege, accessibility to resources, physical abilities granted from birth, and so on. How a person organizes around life challenges is how one can learn and adapt their set of coping skills.

Aiding trans individuals in strengthening overall resilience, ego-strength, and coping skills toolbox starts with assessment. As clinicians are assessing all other clinically relevant aspects of our clients influencing the presenting issue, they should also assess for the resilience. Something that is very common about clients, no matter what they are coming to counseling for, is this sense of defeat for finally coming to therapy—that feeling that I couldn't handle my struggles myself, so I must admit defeat and ask for help because I couldn't figure my stuff out on my own. It's shame. I sense this from some of my most resilient clients who have really been through the ringer in their lifetime and found all sorts of internal resources to keep going despite their painful experiences. This is a distortion, as coming to therapy for help is actually an indicator of resilience and action. And just because a client presents as highly resilient doesn't always make working with them easier, it can mean the ineffective coping skills are just as stubborn as the effective ones. Or the emotional experiences can be harder to access and process due to the strength and fortitude of the "steel door." Clients who might present decreased resilience may have more access to the emotional information needed to be effective in processing therapies. These clients also may be more open and receptive to adopting more effective coping skills that are presented. The assessment of the client's resilience lies within the entire history and narrative of the client.

Nonbinary-Specific Challenges

In addition to several risk factors alerting mental health professionals, there are some very distinct challenges that nonbinary and binary trans individuals face. For example, our society accommodates very rigid and binary gender ideals that leave nonbinary individuals with a minimal sense of belonging. Majority of the studies presenting research about the trans population are frequently biased, providing data about binary transgender identities and leaving nonbinary trans people invisible. Understanding distinct and differing experiences that are similar and different for nonbinary and binary folx, including micro and macro aggressions mentioned in Chapter 3, is imperative to supporting our clients towards gender actualization. To actualize one's authentic self, one must deconstruct the untrue and toxic narratives that prevented actualization in the first place.

Nonbinary gender identities have unique challenges that may not necessarily be experienced by binary identities. The root of these distinctive challenges lies within the binary construction of our society. Our social culture has a high dependency on labels and nonbinary folx often left to fend for themselves. The lack of social accommodation and visibility erases nonbinary identities. Because of this erasure, many people get overwhelmed by the nonbinary concepts, and in response to being overwhelmed they get defensive and dismissive. There is also a culture of public shaming that exaggerates, distorts, and catastrophizes social mistakes, and there are underlying fears around approaching gender diverse populations. In reality, not many people are going to outright shame others for mistakes rooted in not knowing; most folx understand the complexity in this cultural shift and simply appreciate being treated with respect and good intention. Using correct names and pronouns are rooted in showing respect towards another person, and in reality most individuals have good intention and want to show other humans respect and compassion.

Nonbinary folx cannot be reduced to a single gender experience. Expanding upon the material I provided in Chapter 3, there can be the added complexity of multiple gender experiences. For example, there are many people who can identify as nonbinary and also identify with their assigned gender at birth in some capacity. This can be due to integrating gender experiences growing up with one's actualized gender identity. It's a similar concept to the complexity of systems and how people can belong to multiple groups and identities. All the experiences accumulated before actualizing a gender identity can be integrated into how a person sees them self. I have worked with several nonbinary and transmasculine folx who identify strongly with feminism in the way they did prior to gender actualization. Some report that since transition they feel like they have been reassigned to an ally of feminism, and it feels like they are displaced. This is because they no longer identify as women or female, but still live and feel the impact of the experiences they had prior to transition which initially defined their feminist identity. Because of how complicated this concept can be, and how people are generally super uncomfortable with ambiguity, the nonbinary population is vulnerable to internal policing from the LGBTQ+ and trans communities in addition to general society.

There's a lot of intricacy to gender expression for nonbinary folx trying to just live their day-to-day lives authentically. For one thing, "looking non-binary" doesn't really exist for the cis-centric eye. Almost all forms of outward expression (clothing, hair, makeup, nails, accessories, and unconscious behaviors, mannerisms, and speech patterns) are routinely categorized into binary biased boxes of masculinity and femininity. And even these boxes are riddled with distorted stereotypes that serve no gender. This process then results in an internal determination of assigning male or female to someone in passing. Nonbinary people are still somehow categorized as male or female. Lack of diverse representation in media, fashion, and leadership reflect the deeply diverse spectrum of transness. Also, pronouns can get messy as not all nonbinary people use neutral pronouns. This can be for a variety of reasons. Some folx identify with binary pronouns because of how they experience their gender identity. Others find that this practice reduces social anxiety and stress with daily interpersonal interactions. Society doesn't really accommodate gender neutral pronouns in any context quite yet. It can also be for safety because some are just not ready to come out to strangers every time they introduce themselves.

Growing Families

Fertility and reproductive challenges are unique to the trans community due to sorely lacking medical support. There are reproductive opportunities and resources available for trans folx, but accessibility is another gate that is kept by professionals who lack competency or willingness to advocate for trans patients. Currently, the most available options for trans people consist of cryopreservation, or protective freezing of living reproductive cells and tissue. Trans individuals can have sperm and oocytes (egg cells) extracted and preserved; the methods of ovarian and testicular tissue cryopreservation can also be used. The option of embryo cryopreservation is most often performed after in vitro fertilization procedures. These methods are also most available to and highly cater to cisgender fertility, disregarding the medical interventions trans individuals undergo to achieve alignment. And similarly to cisgender women who experience gatekeeping by medical professionals in access to hysterectomies or other procedures supporting reproductive autonomy, trans individuals face gatekeeping from medical professionals lacking competency and alliance. Another primary barrier to accessing fertility care is insurance. Many individuals are forced to take cost out of pocket for cryopreservation due to insurance companies and their refusal to cover many reproductive procedures. Surrogacy is another costly option that is often not attainable or financially feasible for individuals looking for family expansion options.

Medically, there is unfortunately a small pool of research surrounding reproductive options and outcomes for trans individuals. For trans men, if they decide to take testosterone, they can discontinue it to become pregnant, and there have been successful pregnancies. There is also a risk of using testosterone prior to pregnancy as it can impact fertility and potentially fetal development. The current recommendation is embryo or oocyte cryopreservation for trans men desiring genetically related children. Collected from the small pool of data available, for those who used testosterone during transition, the risk of pregnancy and birth complications is also higher. The emotional toll also poses a higher risk for trans individuals' post-partum due to societal stigma, lack of visibility, and isolation (Obedin-Maliver & Makadon, 2016). There is also the consideration of desire to chest feed, as some trans men may want this experience and others do not. Culturally, there is already a lack of lactation support, and for trans men in post-partum this erasure is more substantial. Recommendations are the same for trans women, cryopreservation of sperm. Prolonged exposure to estrogen is linked to infertility, while it is not guaranteed. There have been successes when trans women go off of HRT and wait the allotted time to allow recovery of testes so they are able to produce sperm.

Trans individuals can be processing deeper emotional subjects around family expansion and fertility, and grief is very common for some individuals who want certain reproductive experiences. There are trans feminine individuals who want to have the experience of carrying a pregnancy and grieve the inability to do so. While this potential grief experience is normal and similar for both cis and trans women, there are distinct differences in the nature and context of that grief. There are trans masculine folx who might have conflicting wants and grief. Some trans masculine folx may never have been opposed to carrying a pregnancy, but needed to sacrifice this dream to pursue self-actualization and happiness. Some may feel conflict with a desire to carry a pregnancy, but this need doesn't outweigh the need to remain on hormones or face the social publicity of being a pregnant trans masculine person. The reproductive aspect of family building is directly paired with the body, and aspects of the body that can be sensitive and triggering for a trans person. There are also people who may have grief associated with fertility and reproductive options that may or may not be related to their trans experience because fertility is not a guarantee for anyone. Some trans folx may have taken measures to preserve potential fertility by putting off medical transition goals and come to find out they were infertile later. This subject is deeply complex and clinicians should be mindful of the factors present to best support clients through this messy topic.

It's important to also recognize some positive advances in options for trans individuals. For example, Reisman and Goldstein (2018) published a case report about a single patient, a transgender woman, who wanted to breastfeed her infant after her significant other gave birth. With the help of hormones, she was able to exclusively breastfeed her child for six weeks, and include a regimen of supplemented formula and breastfeeding. At the time of publishing, the infant was around six months old and this mother was continuing to breastfeed and supplement with formula as needed. This advance is absolutely amazing. Providing transgender women and trans feminine folx the opportunity to care and nourish their children, allowing them to bond with their infants this way, grants them access to additional experiences of motherhood that once otherwise would not be accessible. Medical advances and visibility such as these can drastically improve the lives of trans folx who want to pursue expanding families.

Despite strong evidence that children raised in LGBTQ+ households are just as happy as children raised in cis and straight households, adoption for trans individuals is another barrier impeding their right to be parents. There are the financial barriers limiting private adoption and surrogacy options, and the foster and adopt method is riddled with discrimination. Most states are quite ambiguous on what options are available due to lack of concrete laws to protect LGBTQ+ adopting parents, while others outright discriminate by allowing state-licensed child welfare agencies to object and refuse placement of children to LGBTQ+ parents. This information is important for gender affirming providers to be aware of because reproductive options are not truly available and accessible for all people, and even more so for LGBTQ+ and trans individuals.

Reproductive health is a topic that should be approached with care and sensitivity. First of all, not everyone wants children. Secondly, not everyone wants to reproduce themselves to add children to their family. Finally, the provider needs to consider the history of procedures a client has undergone that impact goals for family expansion. If a client is sterile due to certain gender alignment surgeries such as an orchiectomy or hysterectomy, the client has most likely identified their wants for the future family. For those who choose to contribute genetic material, discontinuing hormone therapy is not an easy feat. Discontinuing hormones have the potential to significantly impact a person's mental health due to the hormonal changes that occur, a risk triggered dysphoria brought on by experiencing incorrect hormonal effects, and induced medical side effects. The consensus surrounding recommendations for trans people is prevention, and prevention is very costly, which is a huge barrier for a marginalized population. This also pressures individuals to make very serious decisions about a future that already seems uncertain, and doesn't account for normal changes to one's goals and wants through development. Additional options such as adoption and fostering are also riddled with discrimination and unattainability for many trans folx, leaving this population without many options for family growth.

Being gender diverse already poses specific challenges to a person due to the binary nature gender is integrated into society. The proof of just how rigid and unforgiving our culture is to diversity, all diversity, is in the data. Groups that are not white, straight, cisgender, English-speaking, able bodied, of higher economic status, and Christian, all experience some form of marginalization that leads to increased risk factors for negative outcomes. Being trans is no exception and is often another layer of a person that determines how they experience day-to-day life. The unique challenges that come up in sessions seem to be never ending due to the complexity of not only individual experiences, but the complexity of how their gender identity is received by their personal systems and society. Collecting detailed information about our clients and all possible influences on how they perceive their gender experience is a crucial aspect of gender therapy. Gender therapy cannot really be reduced to and defined by the clinician's ideas about gender; it's extremely fluid depending on the client and multiple factors that define their perception of gender.

Reflection Questions for Clinicians

1 Identify daily social accommodations and interactions that support nonbinary gender identities. Which accommodations do not?
2 How has gender changed through recent generations—The Greatest Generation, Boomers, Xers, Millennials, and Gen Z?
3 Choose three different groups of people with differing race, ethnicity, religion, disability, SES, etc., and list how these groups generally define gender. What are the roles and expectations of men and women? How do these groups welcome or reject transgender individuals—nonbinary folx? Research if need be to learn of the differences.

References

Baker KE., (2019). Findings From the Behavioral Risk Factor Surveillance System on Health-Related Quality of Life Among US Transgender Adults, 2014–2017. *JAMA Internal Medicine*. Published online April 22, 2019, 179(8), 1141–1144. doi:10.1001/jamainternmed.2018.7931

Chang, S. C., Singh A. A., & dickey, l. m. (2018). *A clinician's guide to gender-affirming care: working with transgender and gender nonconforming clients*. Oakland, CA: New Harbinger Publications.

Diemer, E. W., Grant, J. D., Munn-Chernoff, M. A., Patterson, D. A., & Duncan, A. E. (2015). Gender identity, sexual orientation, and eating-related pathology in a national sample of college students. *The Journal of Adolescent Health: Official Publication of the Society for Adolescent Medicine*, 57(2), 144–149. doi:10.1016/j.jadohealth.2015.03.003

Grant, J. M., Mottet, L. A., Tanis, J., Harrison, J., Herman, J. L., & Keisling, M. (2011). *Injustice at every turn: a look at black respondents in the national transgender discrimination survey*. Washington, DC: National Center for Transgender Equality and National Gay and Lesbian Task Force.

Obedin-Maliver, J., & Makadon, H. J. (2016). Transgender men and pregnancy. *Obstetric Medicine*, 9(1), 4–8. doi:10.1177/1753495X15612658

Perez-Brumer, A., Hatzenbuehler, M. A., Oldenburg, C. E., & Bockting, W. (2015). Individual- and structural-level risk factors for suicide attempts among transgender adults. *Behavioral Medicine*, 41(3), 164–171. doi: 10.1080/08964289.2015.1028322

Reisman, T., & Goldstein, Z. (2018) Case report: induced lactation in a transgender woman. *Transgender Health*, 3(1). https://doi.org/10.1089/trgh.2017.0044

Watson, R. J., Veale, J. F., Saewyc, E. M. (2016). Disordered eating behaviors among transgender youth: probability profiles from risk and protective factors. *International Journal of Eating Disorders*, 50(5), 515–522.

White, M. E., Cartwright, A. D., Reyes, A. G., Morris, H., Lindo, N. A., Singh, A. A., & Bennett, C. M. (2020). "A whole other layer of complexity": black transgender men's experiences. *Journal of LGBTQ Issues in Counseling*, 14(3), 248–267. doi: 10.1080/15538605.2020.1790468

5 Transition

Since gender is a social experience, authentic gender actualization is critical to attachment and healthy relationships. Gender actualization is a completely necessary process and transition is co-occurring. Gender identity is a crucial aspect of self that determines social and existential experiences. A potentially relatable example for cisgender people is gender disappointment and infant bonding. A simple Google search of gender disappointment will provide countless stories and message boards of parents who experience significant distress, including depression, due to the sex and assigned gender of their unborn child. Due to our society's heavy reliance on gender, transition offers the ability to live and provides a sense of authentic being to clients.

So what does it mean to transition? Typically, the term "transition" is publicly associated with a binary transgender person, undergoing medical interventions such as hormone replacement therapy (HRT) and gender affirming surgeries to align their gender identity with their gender expression and body. In reality, transition is a very complex and multi-faceted experience unique to each person. Transition essentially means to go across or over, which is quite subjective. Transition is a passage that consists of the voyage between point A and point B. For trans clients, transition is a personal process that is completely defined and piloted by the individual, navigated by their own needs for alignment. This could look similar or completely different between a nonbinary or binary trans identified person. Since gender is a social construct, authentic and congruent expression of gender is critical for daily social interactions with one's internal and external world. It can mean safety, belonging, and ultimately it means being seen as who authentically you are. Finding ways to accurately express one's authentic self to the world is a deeply complex procedure.

It's hard to discuss transition without touching on gender dysphoria. Dysphoria alone is a vague term that speaks to the opposite of euphoria, while in context with gender dysphoria it's defined differently in clinical fields and in the trans community. There are both similarities and distinct differences between the DSM-5 gender dysphoria diagnosis and dysphoria as a personal experience for a trans person. Most descriptions of dysphoria experiences with clients have much more depth and complexity than what's

DOI: 10.4324/9781003001881-6

listed in the DSM-5. There is much more to gender dysphoria than a wish to be another gender; it's a human identity that yearns to just have a chance to exist and be seen. Dysphoria can also be categorized as pathological, which challenges affirming professionals who completely reject gender identity as some mental health issue. Rather, we see dysphoria as a completely normal outcome and symptom of lack of alignment. This lack of alignment can surely be relieved with medical intervention, and for others it's on a more social and existential level. The term and diagnosis of dysphoria is currently an opportunity to bypass gatekeeping and give the community access to medically necessary interventions, which is why it's still used by affirming professionals. We have to play nice with insurance companies to advocate for best care for our clients.

Another important subject to address when diving into dysphoria and transition is the influence of transmisogyny, transphobia, and the romanticizing white, cisgender, and able bodies. Transmisogyny is another layer to the general run-of-the-mill misogyny; it is the cross of transphobia and misogyny. Misogyny is a concept that could be a chapter of its own, but for the sake of staying focused, let's overly simplify it in regards to beauty standards. Misogyny is patriarchal (in favor of men having power), an enforced and ingrained social norm that essentially reduces women to sexual, powerless objects. How sexually attractive an identified woman is, determines how much privilege and worth is granted to her. Most of the time it's running in the unconscious, and other times it can present pretty consciously. Cisgender women have their own actualization process to experience when breaking free of feeling their entire worth is in their bodies and what they can give to a man. Essentially in a patriarchal social environment, sex is power for women. Misogyny not only impacts trans feminine individuals, it impacts nonbinary folx and trans men because as gender context is changing for the transitioning individual, the gender actualization process will be influenced by the beauty standards, sexism, and social norms influenced by misogynistic concepts. Transmisogyny sexualizes the portrayed experience of being a trans woman. Media and social culture perpetuates this by assigning sexual reasons for transition, representing trans women with sexual promiscuity, and reducing them to sexual fetishes. When my clients start dating, trans women suffer greatly. Not only due to severe risk of violence rooted in transphobia, but the constant experience of being fetishized as trans women in addition to navigating impossible expectations of beauty that comes with being women.

Trans women also face transmisogyny through invalidation and dismissal, often by cis women. The sexism and transmisogyny experienced by trans women are frequently dismissed by cis women and trans women are routinely barred from certain feminist groups, known as trans-exclusionary radical feminist (TERFs). Some consider TERF as a slur, others adopt the label, and some use "gender-critical feminist." Though third-wave feminism has mostly integrated trans rights as an important aspect of the liberation of all women and the marginalized, TERFs and gender-critical feminists incorporate transphobic ideas about trans women into their ideology. Essentially, this group reduces qualifiers to biologism or sex essentialism (assigned sex at birth), discounting trans women while often embracing trans men. Trans women suffer in many spaces because of the continued invalidation and questioning of their womanhood.

Something that is routinely touched upon with clients who are trans women is encouraging an early start in challenging the automatic negative thoughts that occur when people stare. Since these clients are women, they will now be constantly gazed at—for their expressive choices, bodies, mannerisms, accessories, age, and potential sexual opportunity. Internalized transphobia can increase dysphoria because of negative messages about one's appearance. If I'm not seen as a man or woman by those around me, I'm failing and I'm an outsider. It can feel like a neon side above your head, and every look you get you fear they see that sign. The notion of the terms "passing" and "stealth" carry the goal of one's transness to not be discovered or seen by the world around you. This isn't an invalid need by any means, while I challenge that this has roots in shame that our culture perpetually inflicts on trans people. The creation and enforcing of strict gender boxes is what we want people to fall into, or you are rejected from the club. For one's transness to be seen is somehow shameful and automatically makes them an outsider.

Three Categories of Dysphoria

For the sake of increasing inclusivity and covering a more comprehensive vision of what transition is, gender dysphoria and its associated transition type is broken into three components: expressive, social, and existential dysphoria and transition. A trans individual will not always pursue transition for all three categories because gender actualization is a different process for every person; transition can be vastly different for nonbinary and binary trans folx.

Expressive transition is the process of authentically portraying the self in order to be seen for who you are. *Expressive dysphoria* can include aspects of the physical self that do not feel aligned with this authentic self. For some, expressive may include medical, surgical, and/or noninvasive physical interventions. I include medical transition within this category because for some, medical transition has a lot of need rooted in expression and being seen. But it's important to emphasize that this isn't always the case, and medical transition is also for safety, physical comfort, relief from dysphoria, personal sense of alignment, and self-actualization. Medical transition is a medical necessity that allows people to live their lives and restore quality of life. Some clients may start varying methods of HRT. Not all clients will use HRT in the same way. Some clients may want to use HRT temporarily to achieve desired outcomes, use lower doses to slow or reduce physical effects, and some may use it permanently while building to the highest possible dosage. Less experienced clinicians exhibit more discomfort with expanded uses for HRT rather than the stereotypical norm: a binary trans person undergoing transition and building up to the best dosage that can be used indefinitely. It is common for binary and nonbinary folx to take different courses with medical intervention as all desired outcomes and needs for authentic expression are different. Same goes for surgical interventions; all trans folx will have different needs for surgical intervention in their transition process. Noninvasive interventions include, and are not exclusive to packing, tucking, binding, stuffing, hair style changes, makeup, electrolysis, hair removal, hair implants, vocal physical therapy or training, and clothing. Invasive interventions include affirming medical interventions. It is not uncommon for clients to experience changes prior, during, or post-transition. The process of actualization involves ever-changing and expanding understanding of the self and what is authentic.

If a client identifies gender affirming surgeries as a necessary aspect of their transition, then this intervention is absolutely medically necessary. The primary options of trans feminine individuals include feminizing breast surgery or breast mammoplasty (known as top surgery), orchiectomy, vaginoplasty, facial feminization surgery (FFS), and vocal cord surgery. Chest construction surgery involves improving the size and/or shape of breast. Orchiectomy allows the person to discontinue testosterone blockers (spironolactone) that can have long-term effects by removal of the testes; though the individual will most likely be on estrogen or some form of HRT for life due to bone health. Vaginoplasty is a genitoplasty that involves the construction of a vulva with existing tissue and vaginal cavity. There is an option of not constructing a vaginal cavity while creating only external genitalia that might be chosen by individuals not interested in penetrative sex or the extensiveness of the procedure and long-term post-procedure care. Vocal cord surgery can be sought to increase voice pitch. Facial feminization surgery can involve a few different procedures, but the goal is ultimately to feminize facial features.

Trans masculine folx have different affirming surgical options. These include: chest reconstructive surgery (top surgery), hysterectomy, oophorectomy, hysterectomy with oophorectomy, metoidioplasty, and phalloplasty. There are a few things that can occur with chest reconstructive surgery. This is can include a chest reduction or a chest removal with masculinizing construction. Chest removal has two options, typically the double incision option is for folx with large chest size and keyhole procedure for smaller and medium chest sizes. Male contouring for top surgery includes different methods of liposuction to remove fat tissue associated with typical fat distribution caused by prior estrogen and puberty. There are also different options for nipple grafting that can be explored between the patient and doctor. Hysterectomy involves the removal of the uterus, cervix, and fallopian tubes while an oophorectomy is the removal of ovaries; the individual has a choice of either or both procedures. Depending on the procedure, this can change the HRT regimen for the individual. Metoidioplasty is a genitoplasty that uses existing tissues to form a phallus; this is formed from the hormonally enlarged clitoris. The labia can be reshaped into a scrotum with or without testicular prostheses. Both metoidioplasty and phalloplasty can be done with or without urethral lengthening, and lengthening can increase risk of surgical complications. This essentially determines the position in which one could urinate, standing or sitting. Phalloplasty uses tissue from other parts of body (such as forearm or thigh) to construct a phallus. Phalloplasty is more in depth due to the complexity of everything involved in constructing a phallus from tissue that isn't already existent in the genitals. In addition to these two genitoplasty options, additional procedures are available for gender affirmation such as: vaginectomy (removal or closing of vaginal canal), penile and scrotal implants, glansplasty (construction or reconstruction of glans), and mons resection (low tummy tuck to remove distributed fat in pubic area).

Table 5.1 shows some comparisons between phalloplasty and metoidioplasty. It's important to note that these procedures are quickly progressing and more options for trans affirming surgeries are coming in the near future. I am also not a doctor or surgeon in any capacity, and mental health providers should always advise clients to consult with their medical providers and surgeons to make the most informed and affirming decisions for their needs.

Nonbinary folx can most certainly choose from the list of medical interventions above to achieve alignment. Nonbinary transition can look similar or very different from a binary trans person, and this doesn't mean anything so don't look too far into it. We are complex and ever-evolving

Table 5.1 Notable differences between phalloplasty and metoidioplasty surgical options

Metoidioplasty	Phalloplasty
Typically less surgeries needed depending on desired outcome, shorter recovery time, and less risk for complications.	Likely multiple surgeries, longer recovery time, more complex, and higher risk for complications.
Less desirable cosmetically as penis size is relatively smaller.	Typically higher satisfaction cosmetically as penis size is closer to average size.
Can achieve erection without additional interventions.	Penile implants for erection ability.
More likely to retain ability to orgasm and overall sensation.	Often retains ability to orgasm, while higher risk of nerve damage that can impact sensation and orgasm ability.
Penetrative sex less possible and unlikely.	Penetrative sex possible and likely with penile implants.
Shorter recovery time.	Longer recovery time.
Typically less expensive.	Typically more expensive.
Uncertain if ability to pee standing with urethral lengthening.	Likely to be able to pee standing with urethral lengthening.

humans that can conceptualize our gender identities differently through our lifespan, and nonbinary individuals should be able to pursue any intervention that suits their needs for gender actualization and dysphoria relief. Nonbinary people have been left out of many diagnostic assessment criteria and standards of care, leaving many unseasoned professionals inexperienced with the notion that it is common for nonbinary individuals to also choose medical interventions to achieve alignment. It is critical for gender therapists to understand that while nonbinary expression can at times seem complex to understand, our culture is guilty of assigning expressive and medical transition interventions to binary notions of gender. Thus, it is our own bias that has the potential to create the confusion or discomfort when trying too hard to make sense of the needs of our nonbinary clients. Don't overthink it and approach this with a gender expansive mindset.

Social transition is the process of integrating one's authentic gender identity into the world. This can include coming out, legal and documentation changes, and integration of identity into family, school, and/or work. Coming out is rarely a linear process for clients. Coming out and to whom are often spread out over the course of transition depending on safety. Typically coming out to anticipated supportive relationships occurs first, and the perceived least safe relationships can occur much later for others. Documentation change timelines are highly specific and dependent on the context of the person. Someone may need to wait due to potential for accidental premature outing to their job or family. Social transition is a delicate and unique dance for every individual due to the barriers and land mines that are potentially around every corner.

Social dysphoria is an experience when personal interactions are impacted by incongruence; it's the internalization of negative feelings when one is not seen by the social community. For example, if someone is not being addressed by their correct name or pronoun, they are not being affirmed for who they are. Cisgender people are affirmed for who they are effortlessly in daily interactions; evidence of this is, if cisgender people are addressed by the wrong name and pronoun (which rarely, if ever, happens) it lacks a potential consequence. Of course, there are outlier circumstances I'm not expanding on because of irrelevance, but ultimately cisgender people do not have a high threat of personal, social, and safety consequences. Once a cisgender person corrects a misidentifying mistake, they will ultimately be seen and affirmed, most times even apologized to. This is not the same for trans people, who have a high probability of questioning, shaming, and possibly even assault. Social transition guarantees safety, not only in society, but for one's sense of self. When someone has a strong sense of self, all sorts of positive outcomes arise from it such as higher resilience, ego strength, mental and physical health, and positive and healthy social supports.

Existential dysphoria stems from the internal world attempting to work out the tangled cords of Christmas lights about who one is. How do I integrate who I was and who I'm becoming? What am I taking with me from this crazy journey and what parts do I want to put to rest? How do I find closure when I still have all these negative feelings, and is closure even an option? What are my dreams now, and what dreams were created to cope with the life I was living inauthentically? What people do I want to invite into my life? *Existential transition* is the internal reflective process of authentic self-emergence; this is the core of gender actualization. This aspect of actualization addresses the sense of self and personal identity that comes into being through the process of transition. Once a person can experience life with congruence, to be seen authentically, they are given the gift of seeking life. Trans individuals are not granted the privilege of congruence because society does not allow gender diversity as a viable identity. This instills a lack of investment in one's life, how can one formulate dreams or goals without a grounded sense of self? Existential transition is the process of learning how to reinvest in life because life is finally something worth investing in.

There's a powerful slam poetry video *A Letter to my Former Self* by Ethan Smith, published on YouTube, that really captures the process of grief all trans folx go through—to release the person they once invested in, the former self. He writes a powerful letter to his former self, honoring that while he made the right decision to pursue living, he had to sacrifice the dreams of the person he used to be. His heartfelt memorial to this former self expresses grief and apology for ending the path of another dreamer to save his life. When I show this video to clients, the reaction is often tears and vulnerable disclosures of their own personal grief they've been hiding out of shame. Some clients feel inspired and will write their own letters, an intervention processed in therapy.

Many clients have a knee jerk reaction to their desire to erase the person they were prior to transition, sometimes because of community policing and way to cope with pursuing transition. Several of my clients breathe a breath of relief when I address grief in sessions because they were afraid to say they were grieving out loud. They tell me that there are sometimes reactions from within the community that police the belief that a person should not have any sad feelings about the part of themselves they are leaving behind in transition, essentially questioning the transness of people who do admit grief. Sometimes it's too painful for clients to deal with all the change happening with pursing gender actualization to take the time to sort through their feelings about the past self and their experiences of who they were. Rejection of the past can help with detachment, and this can be an aspect of the client's resilience to tackle the arduous task of transition. Internal Family Systems approaches from Richard Schwartz can be useful in gender therapy. Parts work is a helpful way to access and personify and externally project the different selves, and it can be helpful in working through existential transition. There's lot to question, how much of my previous experiences were truly me and what was the mask? How much was a performance or role? How much of that existence is something I want to claim and take with me? Sorting through this with clients should be handled from a perspective of affirmation and acknowledging the deep resilience of the community.

Stages of Transition

There are no guarantees or promises for transition; its path is riddled with surprises and game-changers. The passage is rarely, if ever, linear in nature, but it's important to find some sort of structure within the uncertainty that lies ahead. Humans innately crave consistency and predictability because that means there is security, and security is safety. Change, no matter if it is good change or bad change, elicits anxiety so that the person can effectively prepare for acting and navigating the change—with the eventual goal to resume homeostasis, or that state of security, once again. I often compare phases of transition to the stages of change by Prochaska and DiClemente (1983). The stages of change (transtheoretical model) include precontemplation, contemplation, preparation, action, and maintenance. This way, I can provide clients with tangible expectations to normalize their experience. Like the phases of change, transition is not a linear path. New experiences can cause a person to revisit the relevant stage. The concept that phases of transition are developmental in nature was introduced to me early in my professional development by Reid Vanderburgh in his book *Transition and Beyond: Observations on Gender Identity* (2007), and during our frequent clinical consultation meetings I sought with him. The following stages of transition are highly inspired by his work. Reid also writes in detail of the parallel processes of addiction recovery and transition; there are lots of similarities. Using our clinical knowledge of human development and applying it to this understanding of transition phases is incredibly helpful in comprehending the existential changes our clients undergo.

Pre-transition is similar to the contemplation and preparation stages of change. This presents in a variety of ways. I most often will see folx very early in their own actualization process. The client may not understand the way they have felt inside is related to gender identity, or maybe they do have a grasp of this concept but there's minimal understanding of what this means. This stage involves a lot of information gathering and personal exploration in order to be informed what it really does mean to actualize this gender identity. This is a stage where I notice a lot of misconceptualizations and self-imposed barriers (inspired by internalized stigma) present to resist transition or pursuit of further gender actualization. These barriers are part of the person's resilience. In order to prevent change and disruption to one's definition of self and life while keeping some form of security and familiarity present, barriers informed by internalized stigma are placed to keep the person from pursuing gender identity further. I also think it's a sort of mental self-test to see how long the needs persist and how long can it be waited out. This has positive purpose for many other areas of life but can be adopted as an antagonist to opening the Pandora's box of gender actualization. The positive intention of this coping skill is also an instinctual reaction to prevent potential negative outcomes by making change. The brain struggles in differentiating good and bad change; change is simplified as anxiety inducing, and the automatic instinct is to prevent potential threats. Thus, change can feel bad. The ambiguity of transition amplifies this urge significantly.

After the contemplation aspects of this stage are completed, the individual then moves into the planning of how they want to proceed with the new information they have learned about themselves. This is the time when most of my clients sought therapy. Therapy offers a means to gather even more information through self-exploration work, and with a gender therapist the individual can explore deeper experiences of gender to inform them of how to move forward. The gender actualizing individual returns to this phase in some context or another, most frequently through transition, because we are ever-evolving beings who conceptualize ourselves differently through the lifespan; and this can also include gender. For each change one undergoes during transition, there is a revisit to this stage of contemplation and preparation. How we see ourselves is constantly in a state of change until we die, and this can impact our entire sense and expression of ourselves. I guess we can say that the phases of change can really capture many elements of human experience.

Mid-transition is most often the stage of doing. This stage involves the physical act of seeking the resources, interventions, support, and change. This can include seeking professionals to open the gates imposed by insurance companies for medical interventions, documentation changes, coming out to social systems, aligning gender expression with authentic self, and the various other "to-dos" of aligning all of the intricate details of one's life with the authentic self. This stage includes significant adjustment, and gender therapists should be aware that symptoms of anxiety and depression can increase in severity because it's normal to have this response to change—and completely reorganizing your life is quite the adjustment. During this phase, it's also common to see patterns of elevated mood that could cycle with the adjustment distress. While this can be the positive outcome of the client experiencing liberation and coming into one's self, it can also be evidence of the client coping with the stress of change by putting all their emotional investment into the milestones. It's important to watch this pattern because if it's the latter, the inevitable drop will come after the highs of all the milestones. Though this coping skill can be quite useful to cope with the stress of adjustment, it can lead to an emotional dependence on the transition milestones to feel happy.

Post-transition is a time of waiting, but also resuming life and creating the new normal. This is the stage of pause prior to longer term changes or interventions such as gender affirming surgeries. What this stage looks like is unique to every transitioning person because the longer term goals of some folx will look differently from person to person. Some individuals will want to wait to change documentation until they find a new job due to fear of transphobic interactions in the workplace, and others may be waiting to save enough money for interventions that affirm them. This stage can be simultaneously distressing and peaceful, depending on the needs and circumstances of the client. Waiting is stressful and can cause some mood fluctuations, especially when someone is feeling good in one area of transition because they feel alignment, but another area is still stagnant or lacking movement. It can be a confusing time because there are also very positive experiences because the client will feel in control of and invested in their life again.

The *Affirmed* stage is when all the identified transition goals are done. What now? This stage includes many aspects of existential negotiation as the transitioning person is ready for "new normal." The trans individual now has the creative freedom to construct goals for a future they are invested in. After mapping out and pursuing the plan, life just resumes. Some points of discussion might include how to manage coming out in relationships, future family and friends, children, and to doctors and providers. Some folx choose to wear their transness with pride and are open about it, while others choose to drop the "trans" label as they are no longer transitioning and are affirmed as their identified gender. Neither path is wrong. What feels right and comfortable is solely up to the transitioning person. It is not the duty of our clients to be out in order to be advocates. By simply living and being, our clients have battled enough. For those revolutionaries who want to remain open, visible, and seen, it is important to ensure that these individuals have a strong internal and external support system as this is hard work. See Table 5.2 for reference.

Table 5.2 Phases of transition and their milestones

Phases of Transition	Description
Pre-Transition	*Contemplation* and *Preparation*. This stage involves coming to understand gender identity and identifying the needs associated for one's gender actualization process. This stage also involves planning and preparation for one's goals.
Mid-Transition	*Action*. During this stage, the individual is seeking gender affirming intervention, resources, and social support. This is the active phase of transition where most change and adjustment is occurring.
Post-Transition	The individual is finishing up goals and objectives. There is mostly existential work occurring as the individual is settling into daily life as affirmed self.
Affirmed	*Maintenance*. This is the "what now?" stage. Now that gender identity and life is congruent, the person is free to establish what the new normal is and exploring sense of self. This can also be a time of reclaiming personal narrative and making longer term goals for self.

Below are some clinical examples of how gender continues to oppress trans folx when they are affirmed in their gender. These situations commonly arise and took clients off guard as they didn't expect that processing gender is ongoing even after they are affirmed.

Clinical Example

Samantha was six months into transition when she came to session questioning her decision to transition. Samantha was affirmed in her gender at the workplace and noticed a change in how she was treated. She expressed to me that in the years she had this job, she never had issues with her authority over those she managed. Since transitioning she recognized that other male coworkers she managed began treating her differently. While she assumed some of this was related to transphobia, she concluded there was something else at play here. Samantha shared she always heard these complaints from the other female managers but didn't realize how common it was until now. She shared other male managers frequently question and challenge her decisions, they go above her head when they disagree with her direction, and often dismiss her ideas and sometimes later present them as their own. Samantha also reported more questions and push-back from those she managed, including other women! She processed in session that she was afraid of ever having changes of advancement like she has dreamed about because of all the new criticisms she is experiencing.

Clinical Example

Kyle began his transition nine years ago. He was a fantastic storyteller; we shared lots of laughs as he told hilarious stories about his journey. Kyle had a great sense of humor which was definitely a major aspect of his resilience. He told me there was one aspect of his transition that he hasn't been able to get used to. See, Kyle loves children and is quite the nurturing soul who wants a big family one day. He told me a story that once when he was at the mall, a child (who seemed to have lost their parents) ran up to him and began talking to him. Kyle kneeled and chatted with this young child for several moments and even patted their back to comfort them. As soon as he looked up to begin scanning for an officer or concerned adult, he met the eyes of a very alarmed woman who was the child's mother. She quickly yanked the child away from him and was highly mistrustful in her expression. She didn't say a word to him and quickly left with her child. Kyle said that his interactions with women have drastically changed and it's been very isolating at times for him. Women do not trust him now that he's seen as male. He mentioned that smiling politely at women is often misread as an advance and that women seem less comfortable around him when he engages in friendly casual exchanges. Kyle jokingly said he missed his pass to the women's club, as he doesn't feel at home in the strict masculine box that is policed for men.

Another client, Elijah, transferred schools and was affirmed in his gender. He started to notice some struggles socially with his new group of friends. Elijah continued to find socializing with girls easier and more interesting, and since he bonded with others who identified as LGBTQ+, he thought it was a safe space to come out as bi. It wasn't long until girls in the group turned on Elijah. One friend called him creepy after he processed a crush he had on a girl in the friend group. Gossiping about crushes is a very common feminine social behavior, and now that Elijah is affirmed as male, he was called creepy. Elijah was told by this girl that he seemed to be "obsessed" with this girl, when talking about crushes was extremely normal and expected social behavior before he transitioned. Similar ostracizing events occurred surrounding policing of Elijah's social behaviors, leaving him left out of many social opportunities he wanted to join.

Clinical Example

Sage struggled with feeling beautiful. They often processed in therapy that one aspect they liked about themselves prior to transition was a positive perception of self as attractive (rooted in binary gender beauty standards), it was comfortable for them. We spent many sessions challenging beauty standards and deconstructing misogyny, and Sage still really struggled with resurrecting their positive self-esteem regarding this. They explained that all the work we did on gender was great, but it didn't change this feeling deep down about not feeling beautiful anymore because nonbinary expressions are not considered beautiful unless they are somehow sexualized. Sage is correct, beauty standards are a constant daily policing for all people that has spammed advertisements, social media, television, cinema, and daily interactions between people.

Coming out will be a lifelong process. Trans folx will continue to come out to their providers. If the person wants an intimate relationship, they will also inevitably come out to significant others. Some individuals wait to come out to children and others integrate their trans identity into the narrative from day one. A common question clients ask is when it's appropriate to come out when dating. There is no right answer to this. Safety is the number one consideration when thinking about how to navigate coming out in dating. Some people choose to be upfront about it and others wait to disclose, and comfort and safety should be the primary informant on this decision. A common risk in putting gender identity in dating profiles is the risk of transphobic "trolling" and fetish-seekers. For those who want to be more reserved because it feels safe to them, the decision can be quite ambiguous. Just as coming out is an invitation into your life, I often encourage clients to consider that intimacy is a gift that you give those who have earned it. This rejects the notion that trans identities are something shameful to be hidden; rather sharing this is a gift that allows two people to experience vulnerability together. We all have vulnerabilities that we share with people who earn them, and it's truly a gift because these disclosures over time are foundations of trust, connection, and closeness in relationships. All methods of coming out in dating have their risks and benefits, but in the end it all depends on the need for safety and security in each client.

Referring to these stages of transition is not intended to pigeonhole clients and their complex transition process. Its intended purpose is to inform the clinician of some subjects important to explore depending on the stage of change their client is experiencing. Transition is a time of creativity because our clients are finally able to construct their lives around authenticity. Even though there is still work to do with cis genders, majority of cis people have been handed the ability to actualize themselves in the context of gender. This grants a head start in self-actualizing and pursuing a life that fits their identity. Transition can be a time of freedom and liberation for trans folx. And it can also be a time of great internal and external challenges to navigate through.

Reflection Questions for Clinicians

1   Identify how transmisogyny impacts transition for binary and nonbinary folx.
2   How would you support a client who has significant bodily dysphoria but no current access to necessary surgical interventions—both practically (resources and tools) and through talk therapy?
3   What are some interventions you could use in therapy to aid in existential dysphoria work?

References

Prochaska, J. O., & DiClemente, C. C. (1983). Stages and processes of self-change of smoking: toward an integrative model of change. *Journal of Consulting and Clinical Psychology*, 51(3), 390–395. https://doi.org/10.1037/0022-006X.51.3.390

Vanderburgh, R. (2007). *Transition and beyond: observations on gender identity.* Portland, OR: Q Press.

6   Assessing Adult Clients

The diagnosis of gender dysphoria, the fact that it's listed in the DSM-5, is extremely controversial. Just as homosexuality was once labeled in the DSM notoriously, by listing gender dysphoria in a manual for psychological disorders, we are pathologizing an identity; it sends a message to people with normal gender diverse identities that who they are authentically is deviant and wrong. This also causes trouble for mental health professionals because it pressures the assessment process. Clinicians are essentially expected to diagnose an intangible concept: a human identity. In order to adapt to our current socio-political climate, there is purpose to using this diagnosis in the mental health field. In addition to informing treatment for the clinician, it is also used to give our clients access to medically necessary intervention and accommodation. By giving this diagnosis to our clients we are opening doors rather than gatekeeping; as clinicians we can be quite adaptable when it comes to supporting our clients. The diagnosis exists essentially for insurance purposes; this way folx can have access to medically necessary interventions and resources. It's important for clinicians to consider the impact our opinions about the diagnostic process can have on clients; there are institutions in place that we must balance in our treatment approaches.

Formal Assessment

One formal assessment measure that has shown promising validity and application for diagnosing and treating gender dysphoria is the gender identity/gender dysphoria questionnaire for adolescents and adults (GIDYQ-AA) (Deogracias, Johnson, Meyer-Bahlburg, Kessler, Schober, & Zucker, 2007). Some limitations I found with this assessment, and why I chose not to use it, was the binary nature of the assessment and its limited range of gender dysphoria experiences. The assessment can be useful to diagnose transgender clients, not nonbinary, and many of the items focused on stereotypical examples of gender dysphoria that related more to external (social and behavioral) experiences of dysphoria rather than internal. Another widely used assessment is the Utrecht Gender Dysphoria Scale-Gender Spectrum, which has been revised to be more inclusive of

DOI: 10.4324/9781003001881-7

nonbinary genders (McGuire et al., 2020). When I developed my own personal assessment to use, I combined the necessary DSM-5 criteria and the experiences my clients shared with me. There isn't a strong reason I don't use or avoid these assessments, I just wanted something more that aligned more with my own approaches to gender therapy and to watch how specific symptoms and experiences changed over the course of treatment. Using these formal assessments is strongly encouraged for those who find they fit in their own assessment process.

A clinical responsibility of ours is to conduct a formal diagnostic assessment to inform treatment. Even as allies and advocates for the trans population, we still have a professional duty to our license and clinical practice to assess clients. There is no medical test available (at least not yet in 2021) that can physically verify a person's gender identity, we can only go by a person's reported experience. After feeling exhausted in searching through the very limited resources available to clinicians for assessing gender dysphoria, I developed my own method of assessing gender in the initial clinical interview with the client. It is important to note that my assessment process does not aim to strictly categorize a complex experience such as gender, my objective is merely to give myself a potential direction that may best serve my client at the time. The assessment and diagnostic process is about informing treatment, not necessarily about pigeonholing our clients. Mental health professionals often address diagnoses when they are acutely impacting a certain area of functioning. Once the symptoms stabilize, the diagnoses can become a helpful source of information and cease being at the forefront of sessions or treatment if it's not indicated. Treatment is often fluid and rarely, if ever, linear, so clinicians are very aware that the information diagnoses give us can at times be less relevant to what is presenting at any given time.

When diagnosing gender dysphoria, I want as much documentation as possible for the client that evidences their symptoms just in case there could be any future gatekeeping, especially by insurance companies who sometimes nitpick and exaggerate the details needed to grant access to medical interventions. Another intention during my assessment is to inform my next steps. Some clients present with different levels and categories of dysphoria in the initial session. A client presenting with severe body dysphoria may need resources to start HRT before being able to do the intense work of therapy and transition. Another client may be presenting more existential dysphoria and is weighing the options of going on with dysthymia and familiarity or taking the risk to be happy through transition. A different client may need to navigate how to achieve social affirmation and needs to explore all of their options and weigh the potential outcomes.

Gender Dysphoria Assessment

The private practice I work at (since internship) highly encouraged outcomes for monitoring symptom changes. After working with several trans identified clients, I noticed that once their reported dysphoria symptoms began to alleviate, their anxiety and depression outcome scores would also decrease. After gaining adequate clinical and professional experience, I utilized the DSM-5 and consistent client reports to create a scale to monitor severity of gender dysphoria symptoms, called the Gender Dysphoria Assessment (GDA) (see Appendix 6.1). I'm sure this assessment will continue to grow and change with my clinical experience, ever expanding changes within the trans community, and as knowledge progresses about gender dysphoria. I chose to keep the name of the assessment the way it is for now because my intention of this assessment began solely for diagnosis and conforming to insurance and DSM-5 standards; the diagnosis is still known as gender dysphoria at this time. My hope is when gender dysphoria is seen as a medical issue, not psychological, I will no longer need this assessment. For now, it is a helpful and concise tool to help growing gender affirming clinicians with assessment in addition to a resource for clients. I've experienced several clients appreciating the concreteness of an assessment to help organize their experiences and symptoms.

In order to predict the accuracy of my informal assessment tool, I had clients take the Beck's Depression Inventory (BDI) (Beck, Ward, Mendelson, Mock, & Erbaugh, 1961) and Beck's Anxiety Inventory (BAI) (Beck, Epstein, Brown, & Steer, 1988) with the GDA at the first session, and then again sometime after treatment—that timeframe is typically anywhere between 4 and 15 months after treatment began. I found that earlier second-time assessments were unreliable for many reasons. First, since transition is such a huge adjustment and isn't a linear process, the scores on earlier second-time assessment are highly dependent on where the client is as in their overall transition and how they are feeling about it. If there is a setback or an event that triggers high levels of dysphoria, scores will inflate. If the client is feeling positive about their transition, scores will lower. The process of transition naturally has highs and lows, and these highs and lows fluctuate in the same week, or in some cases a day, thus rendering earlier second-time assessment not very reliable for the larger picture of the client's progression. What I did find for beginning and end assessment was the scores on the GDA do go up and down reliably and in sync with the BDI just about every single time and most of the time for the BAI. Clients at the end of treatment might have the same or higher scores of anxiety symptoms on the BAI with lower scores of depression and dysphoria, which is normal due to the significant changes one is constantly experiencing with gender actualization and transition. This state of adjustment is normal and long lasting. Anxiety is a helpful symptom our brains increase during times of change and adjustment so that we plan, prepare, and implement our strategies more effectively.

Figure 6.1 shows outcome measures for the GDA, BDI, and BAI. I collected 24 samples, including assessment scores at the start of therapy and sometime after. Most of these samples had the second sample collected sometime after six months; my collection is quite informal for

Outcome Scores

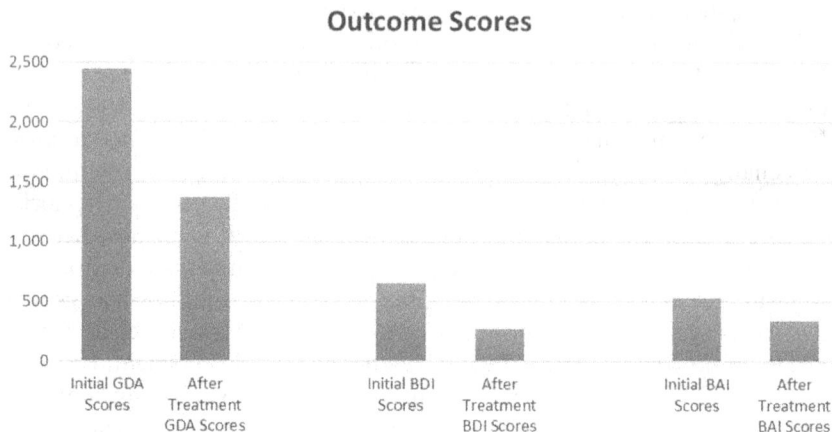

Figure 6.1 Outcome scores for the Gender Dysphoria Assessment (GDA), Beck's Depression Inventory (BDI), and Beck's Anxiety Inventory (BAI) before treatment and after undergoing some treatment.

several reasons. Samples have differing circumstances relating to length of treatment, treatment frequency, personal influences, different clinicians, the pervasive issue of clients not returning for formal termination sessions, and other clinical factors influencing the inability to have formal data collection. The samples were clients coming for gender therapy and worked with me or another member of our gender therapy team. By comparing the assessment scores of the GDA to the scores of the BDI and BAI, we can see a couple of patterns. First, it shows how depression and anxiety symptoms are often co-occurring with gender dysphoria; depression and anxiety scores often went up and down with the GDA scores. Sometimes anxiety scores increase due to anxiety being a natural and necessary response to prepare for change. Second, it shows the GDA may have potential validity as reflected by its use with the BDI and BAI, but I emphasize that proving this suspicion would take much more formal approaches and research that I haven't done.

Spectrum of Symptom Severity

Where a person falls on the spectrum of symptom severity informs me what early treatment needs might be. When referring to intensity, I am not suggesting the presence of symptoms, rather the impact symptoms have on functioning and distress level. After review of the GDA score, this score can inform me of the immediate needs of the client. These groups are not rigid categories, and clinicians are expected to only use the GDA outcomes to support their own assessment process. These groups also are not intended to label the extent of a person's transness, rather the focus is on the type of interruption the dysphoria symptoms present. I am providing examples of what is typical, but none of these groups are absolutes.

Low-spectrum scores, typically under 70, indicate lower intensity symptoms of gender dysphoria. This score can mean many things like person experiencing gender variance has made progress or are affirmed. It can also mean someone has alleviated symptoms after undergoing treatment or has done personal work to integrate gender diversity into their life. In rare circumstances, lower scores were reflected by extreme compartmentalization of gender identity and daily life. Some have asked if this is the range where many nonbinary people fall into and it's complicated. Yes and no. It depends on how someone experiences their nonbinary gender identity because nonbinary individuals can most definitely experience high levels of incongruence and gender dysphoria. I have also had clients fall on this range of the spectrum due to specific circumstances associated with their nonbinary identity such as overall fluidity of identity, visibility and affirmation by society, and personal comfort.

Mid-spectrum scores are usually between 70 and 100 and reflect moderate intensity of gender dysphoria symptoms. Of the hundreds of clients I've met, most fall in this range, followed by upper-spectrum, and then lower-spectrum. Folx in this range typically reflect less mobility in their gender actualization process with roots stubbornly planted in the contemplation stage of change. Individuals in this place often present existential and social dysphoria to be addressed before readiness to address expressive. This doesn't mean expressive goals are not being worked towards or incredibly important, it's that clients in this space usually are wanting to process the "is it worth it?" voice. Clients here inform treatment to address the emotions surrounding accepting the gender identity and to process what comes next and how. Conceptualization and more abstract processing is usually the theme of early sessions. Mid-spectrum persons have specific resiliencies like strong compartmentalization and putting gender identity on the back burner, high distress tolerance, and stubborn stability. There's almost a refusal to allow the gender identity a voice because it would disrupt the flow and organization of the life that's been established. A mid-spectrum client may feel like there are high stakes and a lot to lose by transitioning because they have found a means to cope and find comfort and happiness with their present life the way it is.

Scores over 100 indicate higher-extreme physical and social experience with dysphoria compared to the existential; this is what is referred to as *upper-spectrum*. As I mentioned above, these scores are not meant to be a rule for clinicians to follow since all trans experiences are different, and neither outer-spectrum nor mid-spectrum persons are considered "less trans" than the other. Refer to Figure 6.2 and notice mid-spectrum and outer-spectrum. The pattern I've noticed, by taking this spectrum into consideration, is my outer-spectrum clients tend to need more immediate physical or medical intervention such as HRT and the mid-spectrum clients tend to want to consult for some time before making this decision. Upper-spectrum

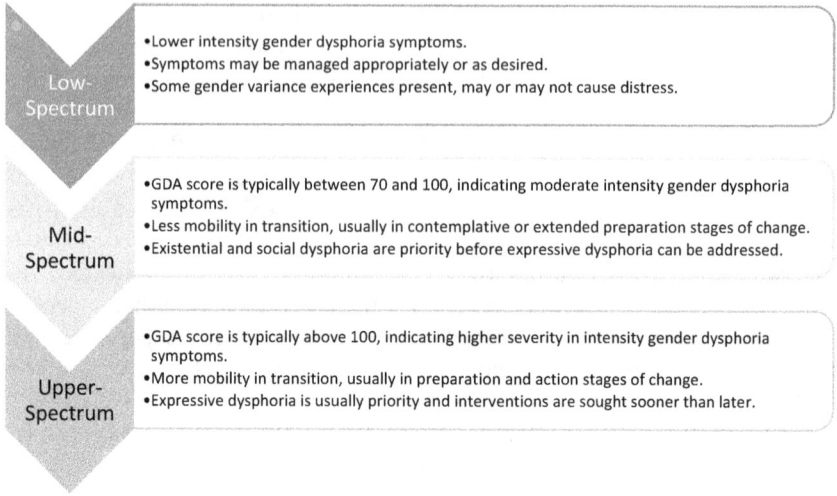

Low-Spectrum	•Lower intensity gender dysphoria symptoms. •Symptoms may be managed appropriately or as desired. •Some gender variance experiences present, may or may not cause distress.
Mid-Spectrum	•GDA score is typically between 70 and 100, indicating moderate intensity gender dysphoria symptoms. •Less mobility in transition, usually in contemplative or extended preparation stages of change. •Existential and social dysphoria are priority before expressive dysphoria can be addressed.
Upper-Spectrum	•GDA score is typically above 100, indicating higher severity in intensity gender dysphoria symptoms. •More mobility in transition, usually in preparation and action stages of change. •Expressive dysphoria is usually priority and interventions are sought sooner than later.

Figure 6.2 Gender dysphoria severity of symptoms per Gender Dysphoria Assessment scores.

folx tend to be the initiators, are in the preparation and action stages of change, and are quite mobile. So mobile, that when gatekeeping stops them, it's incredibly distressing. The resilience of these types of clients is their pursuit of healthy needed change, and as they are jumping in they are really good at active adapting. I also notice that outer-spectrum clients tend to exhibit the most distress and have higher risk levels, making speedy intervention more appropriate. Distress intensity for this group tends to drop significantly after access to necessary interventions identified for their transition goals.

Again, these patterns are not the rule, it simply informs me during my conceptualization and what I reflect back to my clients to aid in the goal and intervention formation process. When I review this with clients, I've received positive responses, most clients feeling they now have a more concrete way to organize their experience and also an affirming way to validate the differences in trans experiences. Many clients have found it informative, affirming, or a dialogue starter.

Due to media and internal policing within the trans community, many clients have internalized there is such a thing as some "level of transness," or a set of rules that determine if someone can legitimately identify themselves as trans or transgender. Because of this, clients have also internalized an idea that maybe they aren't trans. All clients have a set of negative self-talk, essentially internalized stigma, that is a self-dialogue to convince oneself to not transition or they aren't trans. This is a form of resilience, unhelpful at times, used by the brain to try and avoid change because of potential threat. Since being trans in modern society isn't safe on several levels, the brain internalizes stigma to try and sway oneself away from transition. Having the conversation about mid- and outer-spectrum presentations of clients normalizes that there are lots of trans people that don't have the same stereotypical and obvious symptoms. We all know the story, a child who at a young age persisted incessantly that they were a different gender than assigned and it remained consistent until puberty. Many of my clients have expressed a series of doubts in their gender identity because this was not their experience. This experience is actually quite rare—most of my clients report first noticeable symptoms of gender dysphoria being in later childhood, early adolescence. And even then, there are many folx who could not find words to describe their experience. All dysphoria experiences are different. Reviewing this spectrum of the flexible nature of how dysphoria presents has been mostly affirming for clients. Gender clinicians also need to understand the fluid nature of the spectrum if they are going to use it to affirm their clients.

A luxury of private practice is the freedom to adjust documents to be inclusive. I encourage clinicians working with trans populations to adjust their Diagnostic Assessment Form (DAF) to include an affirming gender assessment portion (see Appendix 6.2). The page I made is based on an outline of what I'm assessing for in the first session. Not only will I have the documentation by assessment to support a diagnosis of gender dysphoria, I then collect a history of gender identity development, phase of change and mobility, intention with transition, and present resources and support. One method of assessment for all clients is the timeline method, which involves asking a client to review this history, from birth to now, of clinically relevant and significant events in one's life. This includes family events, important relationships, mental health history, moves/adjustments, life milestones, sexuality development, and gender identity development. I'll also complete a brief genogram as the client is reviewing their story. Having the gender identity development history is an important aspect of assessment as it informs the clinician of all the multifaceted influences on the client's experience with their gender identity. It's also informative of all the adjacent factors that are impacting overall mental health and treatment.

The formal assessment process for gender dysphoria primarily includes the history of gender identity development, the information requested on the DAF page provided in Appendix 6.2, the formal assessment tools of the GDA, BDI, and BAI, and the DSM-5 for diagnostic criteria reference. This method provides the clinician with supportive documentation of diagnosis and informs the clinician of the important and unique information to inform treatment; in this case, gender affirming treatment. This process helps the clinician identify where a client is in their gender actualization process, what resources and support are important for the client to thrive, the systemic influences on the client's experience with gender, and internalized stigma that needs to be addressed. It also informs the affirming mental health professional in how to address additional symptoms that may or may not be directly related to gender. It's important to remember that the assessment process isn't solely about following clinical process, it's incredibly important for clients. Clients come to us expecting thorough, informed, formal, competent, and effective professionals to treat them. The assessment process is important for clients to have faith in the therapists they are trusting such vulnerable subjects with—to give clients a concrete and clinically informed process that they can trust is accurate and reliable.

Diagnostic Considerations, Ruling Out vs. Co-occurring

When considering co-occurring and rule-out diagnoses, it is not a pass for clinicians to assign themselves as the judges of who is trans and who is not. Diagnostic assessment is a very sensitive process that leaves some very clear rules, while leaving some other gray areas for the unseasoned clinician. Gender affirming therapists are diagnosing gender dysphoria based on symptomology for insurance and medical accessibility under the diagnostic code. We are not labeling and deeming people trans and not trans. Gender affirming therapists strictly respect the gender identity being expressed to them. Clinicians also have a professional duty to be clinically accurate and informed, which means we must also be assessing the big picture and systemic influences. Clinically, it's necessary to assess for all symptoms and potential diagnostic influences and considerations. When exploring all the options of rule-out and co-occurring diagnoses, the gender affirming professional has an obligation to be open to multiple pos- sibilities and informing the client of clinical conceptualizations, while also unconditionally affirming the experienced gender identities of our clients. The expected affirming practice is accepting that gender identities are a separate entity from mental health, while the experience of a gender can be impacted by mental health. Some individuals come to us to sort out gender experiences within the context of mental health, and we need to be prepared to balance gender affirmation and clinical duties.

There are some considerations the clinician diagnosing gender dys- phoria should be thinking about. First, ruling out potential diagnoses that could be at the forefront or co-occurring. Personality functioning can impact one's perception of self, and often a person with lower per- sonality functioning can exhibit low sense of self. This can then mani- fest into a higher willingness to engage in high-risk behavior to find the identity that fits. This is because when a person has a lack of sense of self, it can feel like there is less to lose. This doesn't mean that both a per- sonality disorder and gender dysphoria cannot coexist, because they do in clients. Personality disorders can be caused by traumatic experiences, a manifestation of coping behaviors (ineffective and effective) to help navi- gate traumatic experiences. There can be specific traumatic events and/or traumatic relational and attachment experiences. Trans people are more likely to experience trauma as a marginalized population, so this doesn't mean it has to be one or the other—there can be a dual diagnosis. It's also important to remember that the spectrum of symptoms associated with personality disorders are behaviors all humans can exhibit at any point in time without having the disorder; this is similar to many diagnoses that professionals must be acutely aware of during assessment. If someone experiences a crisis, a rough adjustment, depressive episode, or any other experiences that significantly impact the individual, symptoms of wavering personality functioning can be present. When assessing clients with presenting personality disorder symptoms, it's important to provide psychoeducation to clients and assess the consistence, persistence, and insistence of the symptoms. I have met with many clients where personality functioning improved drastically over the course of transition, both with and without the co-occurring personality disorder diagnosis. Some individuals are finally given permission to seek and actualize their identity, which can alleviate symptoms significantly.

Another diagnostic consideration can be trauma. First of all, the myth that LGBTQ+ identities are caused by trauma are just that—a complete myth. It is incredibly rare, but it is possible that trauma can impact how one feels about their body; that said, the rule is trauma does not make trans people. Many would argue that there is possibly already existing fluidity in gender experience that would allow someone to conclude a need to transition to deal with bodily trauma. I personally have not encountered this occurrence; I am speaking to the accounts I have heard from other gender therapists and folx of the trans community. A very small pool of clients have come back later to their provider to admit that certain circumstances led them to transition and they choose to de-transition. When addressing trauma and gender identity in sessions, it is necessary to acknowledge that an incredibly unlikely and rare occurrence and trauma and gender dysphoria can occur simultaneously in a person without being related. How one experiences their gender can be impacted by trauma, but that is something that can occur in all people-cis or trans. Trauma can impact how a person sees themselves and experiences their personal identity, not just limited to gender. It's a complex realm to cross into, and very important for the gender affirming clinician to honor trans identities no matter what.

Similar to the other co-occurring disorders, it's critical to remember that body dysmorphia and eating disorders can co-occur with a trans person. The trauma of growing up in the wrong body, experienced betrayal of puberty, body dissatisfaction, and pressures to achieve certain features to achieve societal acceptance can all be triggers for such a response. Oppression of this population traumatizes individuals with internalized stigma which impacts one's relationship with their body. Body dysmorphia is a rare circumstance when assessing for gender dysphoria, and there have been situations where someone with this disorder can experience distress about parts of their body (such as genitalia or chest).

Many therapists have expressed discomfort working with clients with presenting cognitive or developmental disability and clients with severe symptoms such as psychosis. This is because the therapist is wondering about the client's ability to make clear and grounded decisions that will drastically impact their life (informed consent). There is limited research on this subject, while it is still encouraged to support the gender identity of clients. A publication by Meijer, Eeckhout, van Vlerken, and de Vries (2017) suggests that gender affirming treatment should be given collaboratively with treatment for psychotic symptoms. This is to avoid rigid gatekeeping for an already vulnerable population, while taking appropriate measures to address the risk of misdiagnosis. There has been discussion in the psychological and medical communities that those with developmental disabilities may have had an impacted milestone related to gender identity in their childhood development. Despite theorized causes of gender dysphoria, we must support gender variance and its occurrence in all populations. We must focus on the person's experience of gender and how to affirm it; how it came to be doesn't necessarily matter because there's significant evidence that cause of gender identity occurs in the womb and sociological factors can merely impact how a person experiences their gender. This isn't to say that it isn't our job to effectively do our jobs as mental health professionals. Thorough assessment, psychoeducation, and transparent clinical conceptual feedback are all ways to inform our clients in their journey of their own informed decision making. Determining the client's overall level of daily functioning is also an important assessment to make when collaborating on moving forward. In cases where assessment of functioning concludes to be lower, therapists may slow things down and extend the assessment and preparation process to make sure the client has supportive resources in place and exhibits readiness to make the change. This may also call for more collaboration with family or medical providers involved. All in all, we must internalize and support that the client has personal and medical autonomy. This is hugely why it's problematic to treat gender dysphoria as a mental health condition, it's a medical one and should be treated as such.

Assessment and diagnosis are necessary procedures that clinicians are obligated to conduct. Understanding the core differences between trans gender identities and mental health disorders is crucial. If a clinician has the perspective that gender dysphoria is truly rooted in mental health pathology, it will clearly impact their assessment and diagnosis of the client. Seasoned gender clinicians do a great job separating the gender identity and the mental health symptoms. What do therapists regularly do while assessing and diagnosing cis identified people? Knowing the gender identity helps understand systemic contexts and sociological factors, rarely, if ever, does it primarily inform diagnosis. For example, it's known that cis men typically show depression differently than women. There are more symptoms of irritability, anger, and even aggression, due to sociological influences and expectations of cis men in their expression of emotions. Knowing this distinction is helpful for understanding how gender can influence the experience of symptoms, but drastic conclusions are not to be made based on these patterns. Just because a cis man presents irritability doesn't automatically mean he's depressed. So, understanding elements of our clients separately from the mental health symptoms is an important skill, while also understanding how gender experiences can influence how symptoms are presenting.

At the end of the day, clients have the personal autonomy to make medical decisions for themselves and it is our job to ensure we avoid unnecessary gatekeeping while simultaneously respecting our profession and protecting our licenses. Gender dysphoria should not be a mental health diagnosis, but it is there to help our clients access necessary resources. It would be more accurate as a medical diagnosis that is managed between client and medical provider. Gender identity is a complex and ambiguous aspect of the human identity and experience, and mental health professionals cannot diagnose a human identity. We can however diagnose gender dysphoria which is a set of symptoms and behavior that can evidence a possible trans gender identity. Assessment and diagnosis also provides an opportunity to affirm our clients, to validate the complexity of experiences they are having. To have a structured process, that also retains some flexibility to adapt to the ambiguity of gender itself, is a critical quality of gender affirming therapy.

Reflection Questions for Clinicians

1 What is your procedure to assess for gender dysphoria? Organize it now so that you have an ethical and professional process for future clients.
2 What makes you uncomfortable about conducting an assessment for gender dysphoria? Assigning the diagnosis?
3 How do you plan to manage a client presenting gender dysphoria AND a co-occurring diagnosis? How do you plan to document the treatment plan?

Appendix 6.1

Gender Dysphoria Assessment

The purpose of this assessment is to measure the severity of gender dysphoria symptoms over the course of treatment. Please read each item carefully, and please do not mark more than one number on each scale. Instead, if more than one statement applies to you at this time, circle the higher number on the scale. Noting that symptoms change through phases of transition, please circle the item that best describes the way you have been feeling over the course of the past two weeks.

1. **Congruence**: I feel my gender and my body are aligned.

| 1 | 2 | 3 | 4 | 5 | 6 | 7 | 8 | 9 | 10 |

Strongly Agree   Strongly Disagree

2. **Dissociation**: I feel physically and emotionally present in my daily experiences and interactions.

| 1 | 2 | 3 | 4 | 5 | 6 | 7 | 8 | 9 | 10 |

Strongly Agree   Strongly Disagree

3. **Sense of Self**: I feel like my real, authentic self.

| 1 | 2 | 3 | 4 | 5 | 6 | 7 | 8 | 9 | 10 |

Strongly Agree   Strongly Disagree

4. **Body Dysphoria**: I feel comfortable with my body as an integrated part of who I am. It reflects how I identify.

| 1 | 2 | 3 | 4 | 5 | 6 | 7 | 8 | 9 | 10 |

Strongly Agree   Strongly Disagree

5. **Gender Identity**: I feel comfortable in my gender identity and I express my authentic self comfortably.

| 1 | 2 | 3 | 4 | 5 | 6 | 7 | 8 | 9 | 10 |

Strongly Agree   Strongly Disagree

6. **Future**: I have a mostly clear expectation for my future and I'm comfortable with what's to come.

| 1 | 2 | 3 | 4 | 5 | 6 | 7 | 8 | 9 | 10 |

Strongly Agree   Strongly Disagree

7. **Suicidal Thoughts or Wishes**: I do not have any thoughts of death or killing myself.

| 1 | 2 | 3 | 4 | 5 | 6 | 7 | 8 | 9 | 10 |

Strongly Agree   Strongly Disagree

8. **Mental Fatigue**: I do not feel more mental fatigue than usual.

| 1 | 2 | 3 | 4 | 5 | 6 | 7 | 8 | 9 | 10 |

Strongly Agree   Strongly Disagree

9. **Social Dysphoria**: My identity is integrated into my social life and I am content with my social interactions with others.

| 1 | 2 | 3 | 4 | 5 | 6 | 7 | 8 | 9 | 10 |

Strongly Agree   Strongly Disagree

10. **Anxiety**: I don't feel any more anxiety than usual.

| 1 | 2 | 3 | 4 | 5 | 6 | 7 | 8 | 9 | 10 |

Strongly Agree   Strongly Disagree

11. **Transition**: I am comfortable with transitioning.
It's important to note that transition is defined uniquely by the individual, and
  can be an internal, social, and/or physical process. This response should relate
  to your personal perspective of what your transition would look like.

| 1 | 2 | 3 | 4 | 5 | 6 | 7 | 8 | 9 | 10 |

Strongly Agree   Strongly Disagree

12. **Gender Expression**: I am comfortable expressing my true and authentic gender
  identity in all settings/environments of my daily life.

| 1 | 2 | 3 | 4 | 5 | 6 | 7 | 8 | 9 | 10 |

Strongly Agree   Strongly Disagree

13. **Hopelessness**: I feel hopeful for my future.

| 1 | 2 | 3 | 4 | 5 | 6 | 7 | 8 | 9 | 10 |

Strongly Agree   Strongly Disagree

14. **Accessibility**: I am able to be completely open and transparent about my
  gender identity, or I am able to authentically interact with others as myself.

| 1 | 2 | 3 | 4 | 5 | 6 | 7 | 8 | 9 | 10 |

Strongly Agree   Strongly Disagree

15. **Acceptance**: I have accepted my gender identity as an integrated part of me.

| 1 | 2 | 3 | 4 | 5 | 6 | 7 | 8 | 9 | 10 |

Strongly Agree   Strongly Disagree

16. **Doubt**: I am confident in who I am and I fully intend to meet my transition
  goals.

| 1 | 2 | 3 | 4 | 5 | 6 | 7 | 8 | 9 | 10 |

Strongly Agree   Strongly Disagree

Score Total: _____

Appendix 6.2

Example DAF Page for Gender Dysphoria

Client's Name:
If legal name is different, please identify on first page.

Pronouns (circle one):   She/Her   His/Him/He   They/Them (neutral)
Additional: _____

GENDER IDENTITY INFORMATION
Explain client's description of gender identity:

GENDER IDENTITY DEVELOPMENT
Describe gender identity developmental history:

Does client report symptoms of dysphoria, or marked discomfort related to their
body and/or assigned gender?   ☐ Yes   ☐ No

If yes, list identified symptoms:

TRANSITION HISTORY
Transition is relevant to client's treatment goals: ☐ Yes   ☐ No

Client's current stage of change: ☐ Pre-contemplation   ☐ Contemplation
☐ Action   ☐ Maintenance

Client's status towards alignment: ☐ Pre-Transition   ☐ Mid-Transition
☐ Post-Transition   ☐ Affirmed

Client's status in authentic expression: ☐ Full-Time   ☐ Part-Time
☐ Minimal   ☐ None
☐ Other _____

History of medical interventions to achieve alignment?   ☐ Yes   ☐ No

If yes:

Description of Medical Interventions	Date of Initiation	Notes

Has client identified specific transition goals at this time?   ☐ Yes   ☐ No
If yes, explain:

Has client come out?   ☐ Yes   ☐ No

If yes, to whom?

What were responses like (*positive, negative, neutral, etc.*):

Is client involved in any support groups or supportive resources?
☐ Yes   ☐ No

If yes, list here:

List additional supports client has in place:

References

Beck, A. T., Epstein, N., Brown, G., & Steer, R. A. (1988). An inventory for measuring clinical anxiety: psychometric properties. *Journal of Consulting and Clinical Psychology*, 56, 893–897.

Beck, A. T., Ward, C. H., Mendelson, M., Mock, J., & Erbaugh, J. (1961) An inventory for measuring depression. *Archives of General Psychiatry*, 4, 561–571.

Deogracias, J. J., Johnson, L. L., Meyer-Bahlburg, H. F. L., Kessler, S. J., Schober, J. M., & Zucker, K. J. (2007). The gender identity/gender dysphoria questionnaire for adolescents and adults. *Journal of Sex Research*, 44, 370–379.

McGuire, J. K., Berg, D., Catalpa, J. M., Morrow, Q. J., Fish, J. N., Rider, G. N., Steensma, T., Cohen-Kettenis, P. T., & Spencer, K. (2020). Utrecht Gender Dysphoria Scale – Gender Spectrum (UGDS-GS): construct validity among transgender, nonbinary, and LGBQ samples. *International Journal of Transgender Health*, 21(2), 194–208. doi: 10.1080/26895269.2020.1723460

Meijer, J. H., Eeckhout, G. M., van Vlerken, R. H., & de Vries, A. L. (2017). Gender dysphoria and co-existing psychosis: review and four case examples of successful gender affirmative treatment. *LGBT Health*, 4(2), 106–114.

7 Treating Adults in Gender Therapy

Once the assessment process is completed, it's time to formulate the treatment plan. Utilizing all the information gathered from the assessment, clinicians typically have an idea of what to include in the treatment plan, including the clinician's process goals. Process goals are the clinician's objectives and goals for treatment to aid clients in symptom reduction and the overall progress towards their goals. These process goals are inspired by the clinician's orientation, or clinical lens, to approach treatment. For example, though I am primarily rooted in an affirmative approach, I draw from a systemic orientation, attachment theory and family of origin perspective, cognitive behavioral therapy (CBT), and strengths-based therapy to utilize client resilience. The clinician should review and make note of where the client is in the phase of change of transition and their place in gender dysphoria symptom intensity. Using the information gathered from the assessment about the individual and how gender identity conceptualization could have been influenced by past and present factors, the therapist can accurately direct the client on their path.

While the outline of treatment is highly individualized, depending on both the client experiences and clinician orientation, there are several components I make sure to address in treatment with intention. First, gender affirming clinicians regularly work with their clients to deconstruct internalized stigma. This involves identifying the nature of the internalized stigma and its triggers and responses. A trans person accumulates barriers starting in childhood, essentially negatively biased coping skills that the brain sought out to prevent change; a change such as gender actualization in this current society elicits a strong internal threat response. Because it is seen as such a strong threat, the brain does its best to teach itself to avoid it, thus the construction of barriers that are often rooted in mean self-talk and internalized stigma. Examples I have heard from clients are themed in a lot of all-or-nothing thinking. This type of thought process is exactly how it sounds. Telling oneself that they are considered objectively attractive in the gender they were assigned, so other aspects of life *should* be easier, and this can eventually be enough to create some form of happiness where transitioning is no longer needed. It could also look like mean self-talk that if I won't achieve all the physical aesthetic to make this arduous process

DOI: 10.4324/9781003001881-8

worth it, why bother? This sort of all-or-nothing thinking, almost every single time, sets up the "nothing" to win, and purposefully so the brain doesn't have to deal with this scary ambiguous idea of transition. These barriers are triggered pretty often throughout the process of gender actualization. The brain is highly adapted to try and avoid anything perceived as a threat, and ambiguous change is a loud high alert alarm system.

A common coping skill seen across the board for clients coming into treatment, especially with depression, is reliance on positive life events to get through spans of melancholy, discontentment, or distress. For trans folx, transition is extremely arduous and difficult emotionally, spiritually, physically, socially, and any other way of being you can think of. Relying on positive events or milestones is a default coping skill trans clients acquired prior to treatment. This roots back to the depression and dysthymia experiences prior to self-actualizing to cope with the lack of investment in current and future life. Lacking the ability to be authentic is stifling one's ability to seek personal liberation and freedom. Our clients are shackled by the rigid demands of social conformity. It's common to see clients waiver in their mood depending on their mobility in transition. Transition is naturally composed of high and low points depending on context and its common human behavior to look towards the pay offs to make it through times of struggle. And while this is a common human practice—to rely on the rewards to get through times of hardships—it can risk our client not doing the necessary personal work to emotionally heal. Unseasoned gender therapists might fall into this trap of anticipation with their clients, sort of waiting it out with them until they can start HRT, or come out, start expressive transition goals, or undergo an affirming surgical procedure. But this isn't where the deep healing and therapy is. These milestones are absolutely necessary and critical, but they aren't healing the emotional and spiritual wounds inflicted by negative experiences along the way. Gender therapists need to work on reducing the client's emotional reliance on milestones of transition because the highs after these events are often band aids and distracting from the gender actualizing work. I notice clients often get even more depressed when the milestone didn't fix the emotional needs and hurts.

Transition is a complete reorganization of a person's life, integrating the authentic gender identity into every aspect of one's existence. It's appropriate for clients to formulate goals that align with transitioning, and it's also important for the clinician to be aware that transition goals can go beyond the initial milestones of treatment. Sometimes clients can become emotionally dependent on the highs of milestones (coming out, HRT, gender expression goals, name changes, etc.) and avoiding the deeper processing associated with such drastic and life-altering changes. To reduce emotional reliance on these highs, gender clinicians can utilize several approaches to working with clients with the goal of personal growth and stronger insight. Personally, while I do the standard talk-therapy emotional processing work, I draw from family of origin work, parts work (internal family systems from Richard Schwartz), attachment approaches, and some of Satir's ideas around congruence. I also love to use guided imagery for self-exploration and opportunity for creative therapy. Interventions can range from different specific coping skill building, expressive arts, mindful anchoring in sessions, and other methodical type interventions that entail walking individuals through specific steps and self-exploration. I personally hope to become EMDR (*Eye Movement Desensitization and Reprocessing*) trained and certified in the future to specifically use this modality with LGBTQ+ folx processing identity traumas.

While there may be times in treatment gender doesn't come up, I find that gender identity development and the ripple-like impact of the traumatic experiences are often ingrained in much of the work. For example, while there is a range of attachment styles that highly depend on client context and history, I often see anxious attachment behaviors and patterns in clients due to the pressure to socially adapt one's identity to make others comfortable—the identity chameleon. Also, when a person has a low sense of self, there can be higher dependence on social interactions to provide a sense of worth or validation. Anxious attachment behaviors can have roots in family of origin and be impacted by experiences throughout the lifespan. By addressing this in my sessions, I am not only promoting emotional healing from past relationship ruptures, but I am provided clients with ways to feel more in control and power of their behaviors through gained insight.

Attachment Work

There is a lot in the realm of attachment theory, and here I am going to simplify my personal interpretation of it and its relevance in the work I do with clients. To further your understanding, attachment theory started with John Bowlby, and has had many contributors over the years. Attachment work addresses the client's current relationships and interactions with self and others based on experiences and skills learned through childhood development. Attachment is famously influenced by family of origin dynamics, significant social experiences, and attachment traumas and ruptures. It is essentially the coping skill learned for engaging in and interacting with social relationships. Due to internalized shame regarding one's identity, trans populations often develop anxious-dominant attachment styles to best adapt their identity to the comfort and needs of those around them. This isn't the only attachment style that comes up in treatment, as I've seen my fair share of avoidant attachment behaviors and a mix of the two. Since gender is a social experience, heavily impacting personal relationships and interactions with the world, attachment work is a useful intervention to help clients explore contributing factors to ineffective attachment behaviors to form healthier ones.

There are several contributors to the theory of adult attachment. There are a lot of interesting reads out there on the subject. Personally, I use the four primary categories or dimensions of adult attachment styles presented by Bartholomew & Horowitz (1991), which drew from some of the work of Shaver and Hazan (1987). These dimensions include *secure, preoccupied, dismissive*, and *fearful*. They are categorized based in the spectrum of behaviors and experiences ranging in anxious and avoidant attachment. Both are on their own spectrum from low to high, and both anxious and avoidant attachment styles include a range from effective to ineffective behaviors and experiences. *Anxious attachment*, on that low to high spectrum, includes descriptors of vulnerability, dependence, and higher risk social behavior. In order to keep a positive view of self, anxious-dominant attachment types need the acceptance and social reliance of others. *Avoidant attachment*, also on a low to high spectrum, is marked more by less vulnerability, independence, and low risk social behavior. Avoidant-dominant attachers tend to rely more internally to maintain a positive self-perspective and tend to lean towards behaviors that avoid intimacy (Bartholomew & Horowitz, 1991).

Secure attachment is something most will look for to attain, and even if one reaches a secure attachment style, there will always be some room for triggers to anxious- or avoidant-dominant behaviors. Secure attachment is marked by low anxiety and low avoidance. This style has a healthy balance of independence and dependence, and healthy levels of vulnerability and boundaries. Secure attachment exhibits healthy levels of trust in social relationships and self-worth.

Preoccupied attachment is the presence of higher anxiety and lower avoidance. This doesn't mean someone who falls on the preoccupied or anxious attachment spectrum is necessarily unhealthy; I'd argue many therapists probably are natural anxious attachers under the right circumstance or trigger. We are in a field that helps people; we are people focused and driven by our relationships with others. It's important to recognize there is a spectrum of how high that anxiety goes. Working with preoccupied attachment often encourages an increase in healthy boundaries and relationship expectations. I will often ask clients to analyze their emotional investments and renegotiate healthier levels of emotional investment in certain relationships—to give gifts of vulnerability and intimacy as it's earned. I also ask those with predominately anxious attachment styles to accept the differences in types of relationships and to rely less on social interactions to give a sense of worth or validation.

Dismissive attachment is more avoidant driven, with higher levels of avoidance and lower levels of anxiety—an extreme example, with someone with very low anxiety and very high avoidance, I have referred to as a "bridge burner." Do me wrong once, and I don't need you. Sometimes these individuals appear to not care in their relationships when, in reality, there is a hesitance to take social risks or offer vulnerability because of past experiences that left them more guarded. Dismissive attachers tend to not trust others with their needs or intimate selves. Working with this type of attachment style is typically attempting to increase healthy vulnerability and dependence on relationships that are significant for the individual—to increase comfort with seeking intimacy from relationships. Some of those creative interventions I mentioned are helpful with folx who struggle with vulnerability since it's a less direct way to access those vulnerable and raw inner experiences.

Fearful attachment is marked by high levels of both anxiety and avoidance. I find many clients with this type of attachment style show some immobility and feeling stuck. They desperately want social relationships but feel frozen in being able to do so. Online relationships often feel safer for fearful types because you can have many relationships online, even some that are quite fulfilling, while not having to take many risks since you are almost always feeling in control with online relationships. Fearful types are typically avoiding feelings of rejection and disappointment while simultaneously craving close intimate relationships and not trusting others with their vulnerability or needs.

Many clients express that they don't feel they are changing at all by initiating transition and that their relationships should stay the same. In some ways this can be true, but really an identity is finally liberated that now has personal permission to express itself. While the person is familiar with this identity, others are not. I often explain to clients that while many aspects of who they are may not be changing, their context is. Context surprisingly influences relationships greatly and it's unsettling how much gender matters in cis-constructed social culture. Shedding of relationships is an inevitable happening during transition, and while there can be a lot of grief surrounding this experience, there can also be a lot of enlightenment and recognition of the true purpose those relationships were serving before meeting their end. Many of them perpetuated the trans individual to not seek authenticity or transition. Some of them were rooted in poor attachment patterns and are not very healthy to continue going forward.

Though the shedding of relationships is a frequent topic when discussing human development and phases of transition, it's important to highlight how new relationships gained over transition can perpetuate certain attachment behaviors. Many of my clients with histories of anxious-dominant attachment styles are at risk when entering new relationships. Since anxious attachers tend to depend on social acceptance for positive self-worth, these clients are at highest risk for regression for the sake of keeping relationships. I have seen many clients fall in love and go back into the closet to pursue the relationship because the fear of being alone is higher at the time. Conversely, there can be a lot of distrust of social relationships within the trans community due to traumatic ruptures that have occurred in family of origin and by social groups over time. I see many fearful attachment styles in gender therapy.

The primary goal of attachment work is increasing insight of the roots, identifying how those triggers exist in present time and what they are, and how to intervene. I also hope clients can learn even more adaptability and resist any rigid behaviors or ideas accumulated. Relationships come and go normally through the human lifespan. Just as personal development can be symbolic through seasons, so are relationships. They are constantly changing over the lifespan. Gaining acceptance for this reality, and that all relationships can serve certain purposes and not some all-or-nothing ideal, is a strong indicator of movement towards secure attachment. Through the process of transition, it's also important to recognize the rise and fall of relationships.

Attachment is highly relevant to gender therapy because gender is a social experience. When one experiences the traumatic rupture of identity rejection, this will ultimately influence attachment style because our identities are either validated or rejected by society and our relationships within it. I see attachment styles as coping skills that one adapts to achieve social needs that are often projections of internal desires. As biologically social beings, many personal drives can relate to social interactions in our world. I do not want the takeaway that attachment styles are pathological when my stance is quite opposite. Humans are highly resilient and adaptable, and attachment styles are just that—social adaptation learned by experience. There are plenty of people who lean towards an attachment type and have very healthy social relationships.

Additional Treatment Approaches

Being able to "work on yourself" through the lifespan is a luxury handed to cis people, while for trans individuals, it is something one is finally free to do once gender actualization occurs. If a trans person were to do this self-work prior to actualizing their authentic gender identity, it would threaten those barriers accumulated to keep oneself from transitioning. These barriers are a form of security and safety, the doors to the closet. Trans individuals are often not ready to do a lot of self-work when starting their actualization process because it would release the Pandora's box in the closet they don't want to open. Gender actualizing clients need a therapist who is incredibly comfortable with talk therapy and diving deep by utilizing eclectic approaches that adapt to their clients. Guiding clients through self-insight work is a necessary aspect of the gender actualization process.

We all have "quirks," it's an inevitable part of being human. Through processing work, I highly encourage my clients to radically accept quirks about themselves and their narrative, while organizing more effective approaches to re-negotiate ineffective patterns and coping skills that are impacting them unfavorably. Some of the methods I previously mentioned are ways I facilitate deeper exploration to help the processing work along. Guided imageries are some of my favorite tools. I use one to gather family of origin information and identifying the "wounded child," which has similarities within much more richly complex IFS work from Richard Schwartz. Guided imageries can look similar to spiritual guided meditations that encourage deeper explorations of our more spiritual selves. Some encourage looking at universal and personal symbols to help create more meaning and material for self-growth work. I also use Virginia Satir's iceberg to promote more congruence around experiences with recognizable incongruence. I often gravitate towards this type of inner actualization type work through more creative means in gender therapy. I speculate that the more creative the approach is, the more accessible I am to the deeper experiences of the client. It's like I am given a picture or a story that gives me the material I'm looking for in the process work. My clients have also reported finding these types of interventions less intimidating and more engaging than some other types of approaches to talk processing therapy.

Treatment needs can differ depending on the stage of transition. Social support is a necessary step in supporting positive outcomes for marginalized groups, especially LGBTQ+ populations. Two process goals I start with at the beginning of treatment is ensuring social and/or community connection and progress in emotional regulation to help manage the significant ambiguity and adjustment transition brings. Referring back to stages of transition, Table 7.1 presents some interventions and objectives that might be useful depending on the stage of transition a client is in. Context is crucial, so these guidelines may or may not be helpful depending on the context of treatment. Sometimes if a client likes an organized way to conceptualize expectations and objectives for transition mobility, I will offer them a transition checklist (see Appendix 7.1).

Standards of Care vs. Informed Consent

I will not spend too much time reviewing present published standards of care from The World Professional Association for Transgender Health (WPATH). This is because the current seventh version (latest publication is from 2012) is quickly becoming outdated and the eighth edition is due any time now. WPATH Standards of Care is a document that provides affirming guidelines and a "follow the herd" protection for providers of the trans population. WPATH is involved in advocating for trans healthcare through providing research, publications, education, and involvement in public policy. This association is made up of researchers, mental health providers, students, and medical professionals. WPATH is known for its history in the publication of the Harry Benjamin standards of care. The most recent standards of care, the seventh version, is the standard guidelines followed by all providers of trans care. When it's time to provide letters of support for HRT and GAS, most providers base their needs of written support from these standards. You can find the free document available on WPATH's website for details regarding guidance on mental health support for trans populations.

There is also push from advocates in the field for informed consent approaches to avoid gatekeeping; one of the informed consent models introduced is the Informed Consent for Access to Trans Health (ICATH). Informed consent is different from standards of care. Informed consent

Table 7.1 Phases of transition and treatment approaches

Phases of Transition	Therapeutic Process Goals/Interventions
Pre-Transition	• Reduce symptoms of depression and anxiety. Increase ego strength, resilience, coping skills, and social support. Provide resources and encourage connection to affirming social support. • Help client process decision-making and preparation. Potential guests to attend a session to increase social support and understanding. • Affirming support from therapist and normalizing gender identity as a diverse and unique experience. • Psychoeducation. • Grief work. • Resources for client to begin medical intervention if client has identified this as a goal.
Mid-Transition	• Continue building ego strength and resilience in face of stressors arising with transition. • Reduce emotional dependence on transition milestones and redirect client towards healthy emotional coping during significant adjustment. • Affirming support for hardships during transition. Clinician should normalize client to reduce internalized stigma. • Adult attachment work. Potential family of origin and relationship work. • Challenge distortions and catastrophic assumptions. • Celebrate milestones and process upcoming goals and challenges. • Cognitive behavioral therapeutic approaches to help client cope with emerging anxiety and depression typical of adjustments. • Address existential themes so client can begin process of learning about one's authentic self, and letting go of the mask and performance. • Support for the client reorganizing their life. • Address relationship client has with their community and support.
Post-Transition	• Finishing up final milestones and goals. • Remaining individual work regarding attachment, sense of self, internalized stigma, or other comorbid diagnoses. • Relationships and dating. • Maintenance of progress and milestones made. • Letting go of romanticized perspectives of binary gender experience.
Affirmed	• Address the "what now?" • Exploring questions about disclosure of identity. • Wrapping up any other treatment or transition goals. • Maintenance goals. • Post-transition goals.

Table 7.2 Standards of care vs. informed consent

Standards of Care	Informed Consent Model
Consultation with professional is a requirement, and the professional acts of the gatekeeper to gender affirming interventions.	Consultation with a professional is not a requirement and there is no gatekeeper guarding access to gender affirming interventions.
There may be task requirements a person must meet to access gender affirming interventions.	Therapy is an option, not a requirement, for accessing gender affirming care.
Nonbinary identities are not included, creating lack of visibility or inclusion to gender affirming care.	Nonbinary gender identities are not boxed into binary expectations to access gender affirming care.
Assumes person is not competent to make big decisions about their own body.	Person is competent to make informed decisions about their own body.
Places professionals in charge of assessing and diagnosing a complex human identity.	Does not place professions in position of diagnosing complex aspects of human identity.
Perpetuates pathology stigma regarding gender identity.	Supports autonomy and rights of clients to obtain gender affirming care.

is more about supporting the autonomy of our clients to make their own informed decisions about their medical care and bodies. Standards of care support professionals in a gatekeeper role (while still encouraging affirming care) because standards of care provide a set of suggested policy and procedure that providers should follow to provide clients with opportunities for their care. If we followed informed consent models, we wouldn't need standards of care because decisions would be solely up to clients. The model of ICATH supports that not all clients want or need therapy and shouldn't require an assessment to confirm a gender identity to deem someone mentally competent enough to make their own medical decisions. There is more information listed on ICATH's website. See Table 7.2 for details about the core differences in ICATH and WPATH.

While I lean more towards informed consent in my own practice, I also must consider my license and professionalism and do incorporate both WPATH standards of care and ICATH ideology in my own practice with clients. As much as I'd like to avoid any type of gatekeeping, there are many clients who depend on and prefer the evidenced-based assessment and treatment of trans clients in mental health. The key is that mental health therapy should be a choice, rather than a standard to access HRT, GAS, or other affirming accommodations. That way, trans clients who do not want therapy can access affirming medical and social interventions, and those who want the security of the evidenced-based clinical approaches and want formal assessments and evaluations can obtain affirming care. This would also release therapists from the awkward middleman role that we really don't belong in. Gender identity is a human identity, not a pathology or mental health issue. Yet, we are given the responsibility of diagnosing a complex human identity to get through the significantly flawed hurdles insurance companies have put in place for trans folx to access medically necessary care. Essentially, for clients who do not want therapy and just want the letter, I reduce the amount of sessions to what a clinical assessment takes—usually 1–2 sessions depending on the client. If I am able to conduct an assessment and assign a diagnosis (which we are trained to do) in 1–2 sessions, then that's all that's needed. This is my way of trying to support the autonomy of my clients. If I have concerns from my assessment, I will vocalize them to the client, and I also respect that at the end of the day, if the client has medical autonomy over themselves then they have the freedom to make this decision on their own.

Some questions I've received during trainings or consultations with other clinicians:

> What if my client has come to me with gender dysphoria, but doesn't want to transition due to certain circumstances?

First, I'd challenge the perspective of what "transition" is in this context. I typically explain the differing types of transition rooted in one's gender actualization process, and clients facing this type of conundrum are already "transitioning," or actualizing, by even coming to this conclusion that they are trans. I consider this existential transition at the very least, because coming to terms with one's gender identity is internally transforming the self-perspective—essentially acknowledging that one's gender identity is trans and facing the next step decision. For some, there may be social elements, such as the person having come out to a select few people, which is part of social transition. Gender allies feel challenged by this dynamic because it's drilled into us to affirm trans identities, which usually leads to transitioning, right? This is where we get philosophical about the complexity of the human identity, quality of life, and what exactly is fulfillment. Some may argue that transition has to be the next step for a trans person to feel whole, and in some cases this is not the conclusion the individual comes to. This is where considerations of intersectionality and the client's personal context and systems come in. Being exiled from family, marriage, or even children is a real risk to emotional and existential safety.

So how do gender clinicians move forward with this sensitive situation? Do you end treatment? Flirt with conversion therapy? I explain to clients in these situations that my approach and orientation upholds that a trans gender identity is just as innate, permanent, and unwavering as cisgender identities are recognized; all gender identities are ingrained biological experiences that cannot be changed. Now that the client has come to terms with their trans identity, it's healthier to move forward instead of trying to regress. Trying to squash an aspect of yourself creates major internal dilemmas that will not go away. It will be like a subtle background noise humming in the background. Some days that neutral noise is really annoying for some reason and you can't stop focusing on it, while other days it goes barely noticed. The days it's barely noticed it due to purposeful avoidance and creation of mental barriers to ignore the existential distress (I think of the existential dread meme, don't let it set in!). I suggest that moving forward doesn't have to mean transitioning medically or socially, but it's healthier to self-actualization to at least accept the authentic gender identity is what it is to reduce carrying shame, self-stigma, anxiety, and depression. This could entail processing any grief around the decision to not pursue transition further, or learning to integrate authentic self into one's self narrative. Creating opportunities for outlets, I have had clients attend yearly conferences and keep connections made as an affirming outlet. Do I think this is going to cause the best outcome for these clients? Not necessarily, most of the time these clients come back and pursue further transition or experience more grief for the longing to continue transition. Other clients completely regress because it feels too painful to not transition, and it's familiar and routine to put oneself back in the closet. This is the client's journey and decision to make after coming to terms with one's authentic gender identity. Gender therapists only support the journey of where the client is at. If a client is not at that place to transition, we must adapt and find ways to help combat internalized stigma and shame to reduce mental health distress.

How long is gender therapy? When do you know treatment is complete?

The answer to this is quite subjective and up to our clients. I've known therapists who have mutually agreed with clients to discharge after HRT starts, and I've also known therapists who follow a client transitioning for years and feel stuck. Some clients come in for the mandatory assessment for gender affirming surgeries. Gender actualization doesn't end when this idea of transition is complete. For cis individuals struggling with this concept, think about how one's sense of gender identity as cis male or female changes through the lifespan. As one's experience of self-changes, so does their experience with their gender. Transition and gender actualization are ongoing for the lifespan, popping up in different phases and changes of life. An example for all genders is the experience of parenthood or the dichotomy of gender's influence on self-identity in youth and in age. How one perceives and experiences their gender during these changes are based on life circumstantial changes and phases of life and development. I've had a few clients who do stop therapy and never come back after HRT, which typically is not the norm, but I recognize that many of these clients have done a lot of self-work to prepare for journeying through the process without therapy. Others simply do not have the resources, desire and commitment, or trust to continue therapy. Some stop too early, getting fooled by the "high" of the milestones I discussed earlier in this chapter.

So, when does gender treatment end? Most times I rely on the client to inform me of this. Outcomes are looking good (assessment measure outcomes and treatment plan outcomes), client has maintained stable progress and mood, and client is highly familiar and utilizing important resources. As with all clients, sometimes we find clients are hesitant to end the therapeutic relationship due to the strong impact on their lives. For trans folx, a therapist can be even more, like the first person they came out to, the first person to affirm and see them, and the safest space they can be raw and honest about themselves. It's a scary thing to move on from. I encourage stepping down first and reducing frequency for clients struggling with ending treatment. Then, when it comes time to terminate, I offer post-treatment consultation sessions or a reminder they can reach out in the future. Post-treatment consultations are 1–3 sessions a client can use to come back without re-engaging in the entire treatment process. It's more about checking in and consulting about a specific trigger or issue that arises without restarting treatment. Many clients like this option, and it's not unusual for me to hear from a client several years later to either return to treatment for a little bit around a specific issue or for post-treatment sessions. This has helped many with the transition out of treatment, allowing clients to test their growth.

Treatment ends when there are no treatment goals left, when the client feels integrated and affirmed in their gender, and when they are practically prepared to move forward without therapy. Sometimes, if there are comorbid symptoms outside of my specialty, a referral is next—maybe EMDR for trauma or DBT for emotional regulation struggles not resolved through gender therapy and treatment with me. It's highly important the client has social supportive resources upon discharge. Not only is this important for clients of all clinical populations, but for trans folx, being seen and affirmed is crucial.

> How do I even write an HRT or GAS letter of support for my client? This seems like a tricky letter to write and I'm nervous.

There are a lot of providers working with trans folx who are afraid of liability. Some of this is internalized by our education, professional standards, and tension in our socio-political climate where providers are often one of the first blamed when something deemed mental health related goes awry. Because of this, letter writing tends to be the primary consultation topic I get. I have provided examples in Appendices 7.2 and 7.3 of HRT and GAS support letter structure I typically use. I will also stress that details of these letters heavily depend on context, and sometimes I get push back from insurance companies and surgeons and must adapt my letters. This is just a basic structure I am providing, and I encourage any provider using it to adapt their letters to their own professional style. The standard advice I provide in these situations is NEVER go beyond your competence. It is very easy for a provider to want to go a step further out of pressure or desire to help our clients. This is where there is a risk spectrum of liability. I once had a question from a clinician asking if it would be okay to speak to a person's medical need for a hysterectomy due to chronic pain for endometriosis; this was within the same letter for surgery to alleviate gender dysphoria. First, we cannot speak to medical diagnoses and needs, we are only strictly able to speak to mental health needs. Secondly, therapists are only writing letters relevant to the gender dysphoria diagnosis in these cases. We must strictly word our letters to reflect our scope.

There is also sometimes push back from surgeons or insurance companies asking us to include information we cannot provide, so don't provide it. What we can do is find ways to try and touch on subjects necessary for insurance to cover the surgeries if we can. Using statements "to my knowledge" or "per client's report" are useful. So, there are real practical ways clinicians can avoid gatekeeping from fear of writing letters. There is a lot of room for creativity in support letter writing to help alleviate liability fears, while supporting clients. If the provider can formally assess and diagnose a client, they most definitely can and should write these letters of support for medically necessary interventions that will alleviate the pain and suffering of our clients.

For seasoned gender clinicians, there is a resource available to the public that is worth consideration. The Gender Affirming Letter Access Project (GALAP) is made up of a group of mental health professionals who support the agency of trans folx and the informed consent model for accessing affirming medical intervention. I have recently found out about this project and signed up. Many of us are busy and thinking about how pro-bono services can be overwhelming depending on the stage of our professional development, and what I appreciate about this project is that clinicians can simply commit to providing one letter and session a month, pro-bono, to contribute to the advocacy work. For clinicians comfortable with the assessment and letter writing process, this is a great opportunity to give back and advocate for the medical autonomy of the trans community.

> I am a counselor located in a rural area where there is no ability to refer to specialists. What should I do when I get a referral for gender therapy?

Rural counselors must rely on a different set of resources than counselors located within proximity to cities and more populated areas. Rural counselors also have a lot of pressure to provide services for a wide array of client needs which makes it incredibly difficult, nearly impossible, to specialize. Unfortunately, since many of us were not given this sort of education during our programs, it falls on the providers to seek at least a minimum of foundational gender 101 information to mitigate harm to gender therapy clients. Trainings and consultations for learning foundational concepts of being affirming are quite assessable through a quick internet search. There are lots of available video or in-person trainings found through continuing education (CEU) providers and community organizations. There are also many gender therapy experts available for consultation and supervision via phone or videocall, and this could be a valuable resource and a feasible option. I consulted with a retired gender therapist for two years every month while I built my specialty.

In addition to the expectation that rural clinicians, at absolute minimum, learn basics of being affirming, informed consent and provider transparency goes a long way. It is best practice for all mental health providers to inform clients of the scope of their clinical competency and experience. Tell the client what you can help with and what you might not be able to help with. Inform them when you are going to seek consultation about a particular issue you aren't familiar with. This kind of upfront information will allow the client the autonomy to choose next steps and empower them to have leadership in their treatment. If the client chooses to continue with a provider less informed in gender therapy, a strong rapport and therapeutic alliance will be critical in going forward.

Finally, my advice for rural counselors is to avoid being a gatekeeper. If you can diagnose a client, you can give the diagnosis of gender dysphoria. If you can diagnose a client with gender dysphoria, you can write a letter of support so the client can have access to medically necessary interventions. If this is an uncomfortable practice, have resources or referrals prepared and available, or seek the support you need to become more comfortable.

Below are some resources I've used or given to clients and other providers. Some of these organizations provide training, resources, or reading material to increase awareness and education. Others are advocacy projects that could be helpful to get involved with or become more aware of.

American Counseling Association (ACA)
American Psychological Association (APA)
Black Trans Advocacy Coalition (BTAC)
COLAGE
GALAP
GATE
Gender Diversity
Gender Spectrum
GLAAD
GLSEN
Human Rights Campaign (HRC)
LGBT Foundation
The National Center for Trans Equality
The Okra Project
PFLAG
REFUGE
Silvia Rivera Project
SPART*A
The Youth & Gender Media Project
Transgender American Veterans Association

Trans Athletes.com
Trans Latina Coalition (TLC)
Transgender Law Center
Trans People of Color Coalition (TPCC)
Trans Student Educational Resources (TSER)
Trans Women of Color Collective (TWCC)
Trans Youth Family Allies
Trans Youth Equality Foundation
The Trevor Project
World Professional Association for Transgender Health (WPATH)

Reflection Questions for Clinicians

1   Think about your personal clinical approaches and favorite interventions and inspirations for your work. How can you adapt them to help a client actualize themselves and gender identity?
2   What scenario might you have second thoughts in providing a letter of support for a client (this isn't limited to gender therapy). What is the theme or context of your discomfort, and is there any room within your professional decision to provide this for your client?
3   How might you explore attachment with clients? What interventions can be used to explore family of origin and relationship patterns?

Appendix 7.1

Transition Checklist

Pre-Transition Goals	
☐	Conduct personal research and exposure to appropriate information to help decision-making and goal planning process
☐	Contact mental health professional to begin transition and actualization process
☐	Seek external affirmative resources: support groups, online communities, etc.
☐	Begin coming out process
☐	Create brief timeline for short-term and/or long-term transition goals
My Social Transition Goals (includes coming out and social integration)	
☐	
☐	
☐	

☐	
☐	
☐	
☐	
☐	
☐	
☐	

My Gender Expression Transition Goals (invasive and noninvasive objectives)

☐	
☐	
☐	
☐	
☐	
☐	
☐	
☐	
☐	
☐	

My Existential Transition Goals (identity, emotional health, personal growth)

☐	
☐	
☐	
☐	
☐	
☐	
☐	
☐	
☐	
☐	

	Pre-HRT Checklist (if applicable)
☐	Reproductive decision-making (preserving/storing eggs or sperm? Adoption, fostering, or no children option?)
☐	Research and/or consult about HRT and establish concrete goals for HRT treatment
☐	Conduct analysis and planning of financial obligations for transition goals, including review of insurance benefits
☐	Contact HRT-providing physician
☐	Undergo assessment and obtain letter from mental health professional (if this is still necessary in your area)
☐	Begin building wardrobe and/or makeup, accessories, and other affirming gender expressive tools
☐	
☐	
	School Checklist (if applicable)
☐	Meet with school counselor and/or administrative staff to address transition at school
☐	Complete gender and transition support plans with school staff
☐	Come out to appropriate staff to begin integrating name and pronoun at school
☐	Engage supportive resources (Gay Straight Trans Alliance [GSTA], etc.)
☐	Plan for comfortable and appropriate bathroom use
☐	Plan for reporting any harassment or bullying
☐	Obtain updated ID (preferred name and pronoun, gender marker, email, badge, directory, uniforms, etc.)
☐	Come out to peers
☐	Go full-time
☐	
☐	
	Work Checklist (if applicable)
☐	Research or review policy in the workplace and create plan accordingly
☐	Come out to diversity specialist or HR, express intent to transition in the workplace
☐	Come out to boss and/or supervisor, expressing intent to transition

☐	Create plan for transition in the work place, collaborating with management staff
☐	Encourage educational resources for management if indicated
☐	Come out to peers according to plan created with management team
☐	Obtain updated ID (preferred name and pronoun, gender marker, email, badge, directory, uniforms, etc.)
☐	Inform appropriate staff of any updated legal documents
☐	Plan for comfortable and appropriate bathroom use
☐	Plan for reporting any harassment in the workplace
☐	Go full-time at work
☐	
☐	

Documentation Checklist	
☐	Legal name change
☐	BMV name change and gender marker change
☐	Birth certificate (if applicable)
☐	Social security card
☐	Passport
☐	Utility accounts name change (electric, water, rent/home documents, phone bill, trash, etc.)
☐	Insurance policies name change
☐	Other I name changes (military, work, school, etc.)
☐	Financial and bank accounts name change (retirement accounts, loans, mortgage, etc.)
☐	Degree and diploma updates
☐	Wills and power of attorney
☐	Marriage certificate
☐	Assets ownership documents
☐	
☐	

Appendix 7.2

Sample of HRT Letter

Clinician Name and Credentials
Address
Phone

Doctor or Staff Name
Address
Phone
Fax

Date

To whom it may concern

This letter is with regards to *client's identified name* (Legal name if applicable and DOB). I have attached a copy of the release of information I have obtained from *client* to communicate with you about this case.

I am currently *client's* mental health provider for counseling services at *Practice/ Agency Name*. As a part of their process for gender actualization, *client* began therapy on *start date*. *Client* has attended *number of sessions* and we have discussed the plan for transition and continuing with therapy as a means to address any issues that may arise during their transition process. *Client* meets criteria for the diagnosis of Gender Dysphoria per client's reported symptoms meeting DSM-5 diagnostic criteria. *Client* reports consistent discomfort with the incongruence of their gender identity and assigned body and has made the decision to initiate hormone therapy in order to better align their gender with their body.

I am referring this client to you for consultation for possible hormone replacement therapy. Please feel free to contact me at—put your information here—if there are any further questions regarding this client.

Sincerely,

Caitlin Yilmazer, MA, LPCC-S
Licensed Professional Clinical Counselor

Appendix 7.3

Sample of GAS Letter

Clinician Name and Credentials
Address
Phone

Doctor or Staff Name
Address
Phone
Fax

Date

To whom it may concern

This letter is with regards to *client's identified name* (Legal name if applicable and DOB). I have attached a copy of the release of information I have obtained from *client* to communicate with you about this case.

I am currently *client's* mental health provider for counseling services at *Practice/ Agency Name*. *Client's* focus of treatment is reaching personal congruence by aligning and integrating their gender identity in their life. *Client* exhibited the following symptoms of gender dysphoria according to DSM-5 criteria: (1) a marked incongruence in experienced gender and sex characteristics, (2) a strong desire to be rid of sex characteristics because of the marked incongruence with experienced gender, (3) a strong desire for the sex characteristics of another gender, (4) a strong desire to be another gender, (5) a strong desire to be treated as another gender, and (6) a strong conviction that they have the typical feelings and reactions of another gender. *Client* has reported a history of clinically significant symptoms of gender dysphoria and has initiated the transition process, reaching personal goals (*including goals and objectives that were identified and met by client*). "*If applicable add here: Client resolved/is managing coexisting diagnose of … over the course of treatment*" OR "*client's coexisting symptoms of anxiety and depression are directly related to their experience with gender dysphoria.*"

As a part of their process for gender actualization, *client* began therapy on *first session date*, and has attended *number of sessions. Include identified and met goals by client, for example*: *Client* has been living as their authentic gender for six months and has been on HRT for one year. *Client* reports consistent discomfort with their body and has made the decision to initiate Gender Affirming Surgery (GAS) in order to better align their gender identity with their body. Client reports intent to pursue *insert surgical intervention here* to alleviate symptoms of gender dysphoria.

Edit this paragraph with evidence of gender dysphoria from treatment: I am confident that *client* is practically prepared to live as their intended gender post-transition, as evidenced by their report during treatment. *Client* has completed treatment goals related gender actualization and addressing any challenges they may face post transition. *Client* has reported making necessary steps towards personal and treatment goals, such as: living as their intended gender, reducing intrusive symptoms of gender dysphoria, accessing appropriate and supportive resources, and strengthening their supportive relationships. Client is also an active advocate for the community and regularly attends support group. This evidence indicates *client's* readiness to live as their intended gender successfully post-surgery.

According to WPATH standards of care, *client* meets necessary criteria indicating readiness for medical intervention. My awareness of met criteria is based on client's report of: persistent symptoms of gender dysphoria, preparedness to make a fully informed decision and consent for treatment, and their ability to reasonably manage symptoms congruent with gender dysphoria. Per *client's* report, *client* has reasonable expectations and an understanding of the process undergoing *surgical intervention* and is capable to make an informed decision about initiating this intervention. To my knowledge, from *client's* report, *client* has sought consultation with appropriate medical professionals about addressing any existing medical issues, and the only presenting mental health symptoms are related to gender dysphoria.

I hope this information is beneficial in helping determine the best ongoing care for my client. Please feel free to contact me at—*put your information here*—if there are any further questions regarding this client.

Sincerely,

Caitlin Yilmazer, MA, LPCC-S
Licensed Professional Clinical Counselor

References

Bartholomew, K., & Horowitz, L. M. (1991). Attachment styles among young adults: a test of a four-category model. *Journal of Personality and Social Psychology*, 61, 226–244.

Hazan, C., & Shaver, P.A. (1987). Romantic love conceptualized as an attachment process. *Journal of Personality and Social Psychology*, 52, 511–524.

8 Assessment and Treatment of Gender Diverse Children and Teens

From an affirmative lens, gender identities are innate and biological, a permanent aspect of a person's being. This concept doesn't change when working with gender nonconforming children and teens. But what *can* change is the expression or experience of a gender. Children as young as two years old have been documented exhibiting symptoms of gender dysphoria. What does this even look like? The thought of a two-year old with the cognitive capacity to make such conclusions tends to elicit anxiety, defensiveness, and doubt in our society. This chapter will explore gender identity development for gender nonconforming children spanning to trans teens, providing clinicians information about the assessment process. While there are many similarities in working with trans teens and adults, there are important unique circumstances to be considered, explored, and addressed. The examples I provide in this chapter are purposefully exaggerated and stereotypical for the sake of comprehension and applicability. All stories are different and unique, and more often stories will contain vague recollections and subtle symptoms of gender dysphoria because all people conceptualize identity differently.

Gender Diverse Children

Not all trans and gender nonconforming teens and adults exhibited signs or symptoms of gender dysphoria in early childhood. Despite the focused media attention of these narratives, it has been in my clinical experience that most of my trans clients report beginning to notice and exhibit signs between the ages of 9 and 14 years. This could be due to a variety of reasons. The intensity and nature of the dysphoric experience is unique to every individual, which may cause some folx to express gender dysphoria at younger or older ages. It could relate to family culture and how rigid or fluid gender expression is in the household, influencing how quickly or later the child can perceive and conceptualize their experience. It can also relate to puberty, as the incongruence in gender and body experience. There are no transgender children, they are considered gender nonconforming, gender variant, or gender diverse until adolescence. This is because, while some gender nonconforming children will grow and be trans, many will

DOI: 10.4324/9781003001881-9

not, and they are simply in the process of understanding their gender identity. Gender nonconforming behavior is a common experience for gender diverse *and* cisgender children, and studies are very conflicted with regard to correlations in childhood expressions of gender variance being predictors for future trans identity.

One strong predictor is the intensity of gender dysphoria in children, but I emphasize that this evidence should not be the primary assessment. This is because the intensity of gender dysphoria is not the only predictor of a person's future gender identity, as most of my clients do not report intense gender dysphoria from young childhood. This information is meant to be used as psychoeducation for the clinician and family that if a child is presenting severe gender dysphoria, there is correlation to consistent gender diverse identity. The primary informal assessment I fall back on is the collection of symptoms and their relationship to consistence, persistence, and insistence. If these three indicators are present through the history of symptoms in the child and they meet DSM-5 and WPATH assessment criteria, I assign the diagnosis of gender dysphoria in childhood.

Kristina Olson of the University of Washington is the founder of the TransYouth project, which is currently undertaking the largest US-based longitudinal study for gender nonconforming children, following about 300 children for 20 years; the study began in 2013. So far, the information gathered is showing a strong indication that trans children who have socially transitioned show very similar patterns of gender development as cisgender children. Many of these children are also showing positive mental health outcomes with the support of their families. As part of this developing longitudinal study, a publication from 2019 (Rae et al., 2019) followed 85 children ranging from 3 to 12 years old exhibiting gender diversity. They were followed up with two years later, and of the 85 children, 36 had so far socially transitioned. This reflects consistence, persistence, and insistence of gender dysphoria, which is the primary assessment tool gender therapists use in assessing gender nonconforming children.

Clinical Example

Nicole is a five-year-old gender nonconforming child who started showing signs of gender nonconformity between two and three years of age. Her family came to a few sessions to consult with me about how to best support her going forward. Nicole's earliest signs began when she started to speak. Her parents informed me that Nicole would correct her parents from a very young age, insisting she was a girl and not the boy they referred to her as; she has even kept the name that she gave herself! Nicole was showing severe signs of anxiety in her outbursts and irritability at school and her parents began to worry about her emotional wellbeing. She was hiding under tables and chairs and hitting and biting other children who referred to her as a boy. They told me that Nicole would become another child at school, and when she was home and could wear dresses, she was an extroverted, relaxed, and happy child. It wasn't until she told her mother earlier that year that she didn't want to live if she had to grow up to be a boy that her parents began to understand this wasn't just play for Nicole.

The child in this example exhibits gender nonconformity and is diagnosed with gender dysphoria—what are the next steps? When working with children, I've found that children are typically happier and well-adjusted once their parents, family, and community affirm and support them. Much of my work is with the parents to provide psychoeducation, resources, therapeutic support for grief emotions and emotional processing, and collaborating on how to be a liaison for the child with school, community, and family. Working with transitioning families is a huge aspect of working with gender nonconforming minors, especially children. The stages for these families are presented in Chapter 9 and can be a useful tool to explore with parents during the psychoeducational and therapeutic aspects of work with them. Social transition is the primary way to support the child, and this looks different for all children depending on how their identity is experienced and the intensity of dysphoria. Social transition for a child can include changes in name and pronoun, wardrobe, hair style, and social accommodations. This can be very hard on the parents and family because not only are they trusting a younger child to take the lead on a huge life change (it can feel counterintuitive and conflicting for parents), but the family is most likely grieving. It doesn't matter how supportive and affirming a parent is, they will grieve. In our current society, it's impossible not to have attachments to gender. It has to do with the bonding and context of a child for many people. Grief is normal and expected because it's a huge change with very uncertain outcomes. The ambiguity of the future and how the child will identify can be crushing for many parents because knowing their gender identity feels like a foundational aspect of bonding and connection in the parent–child relationship.

A very helpful resource I encourage parents to utilize is the Gender Support Plan provided by Gender Spectrum (www.tfaforms.com/4745264); this resource is highly valuable. The Gender Support Plan Gender Spectrum provides is best used in a meeting between family and appropriate school staff (such as a school guidance counselor or administrator who handles student support). This document allows the family and gender diverse child to establish the expectations and needs from the school to support the developing gender of the child. The document not only supports the child or teen, but it's a document that can protect the school since there's a concrete plan in place to avoid liability. This form can be used to assess all ages of students.

Prepubescence

Clinical Example

Grayson was ten when he began to realize the incongruence in how he felt about himself and how others saw him. He always felt like "one of the guys" and enjoyed playing football with his brothers and their friends. It hadn't yet clicked for him when his mother told him to stop going outside without his shirt on. None of these clues really occurred to him until his mother sat down and taught him about menstruation and puberty. While this talk is terrifying for many pre-pubescent children, Grayson developed severe anxiety and dread. He would cry at the thought of developing a feminine chest or birthing a child one day. He preferred masculine clothing and began wearing baggy clothes to hide his body, telling his parents that he hated his body and felt like it was betraying him.

Prepubescence is the most common phase of development where my clients identify early experiences of gender nonconformity. Puberty can be a physically traumatizing experience and the incongruence between body and gender identity is becoming more apparent and distressing. This is also a delicate time for the child and families as they try and grapple with the decision to initiate puberty suppressants. Medical intervention is not a possibility for gender nonconforming children, but for prepubescent gender diverse kids, the decision to consult about hormone blockers, or puberty suppressing medication, is on the horizon. Consulting with medical specialists is my recommendation to families, and luckily my resource is the Children's Hospital Transgender Health Clinic, a highly specialized resource for families and trans minors. Puberty suppressants have been used for a long time; its history has roots in delaying puberty for early menstruating children. Many medical professionals believe the psychological effects of puberty of the wrong gender are more severe than the potential mild effects of trying a puberty suppressant because the physiological changes of puberty are not reversible. Puberty suppressants buy time, and if the child does not want to transition, once they stop the blockers, they start puberty. I stress to my families that I am not a medical provider, and detailed discussion and assessment should be conducted with a specialized medical provider.

Treatment for prepubescent gender nonconforming children is like younger children. The primary difference is the decision-making process of how to move forward with affirming the child. The child typically has more skills to convey what they are experiencing and need going forward, so the gender therapist needs to facilitate this in individual and family sessions. Psychoeducation will also extend to the child so they can better understand physiological changes with or without hormonal intervention and holding space to process these decisions and changes. Prepubescent gender diverse children tend to be overall well-adjusted when they are being affirmed at home and in their communities, much like younger children, but their emotional processing abilities are increasing. Clinicians should be prepared to meet their developing verbal and emotional processing skills and explore concepts surrounding self-actualization through the context of their authentic gender.

Adolescence

Clinical Example

Sam is a 16-year-old nonbinary person who came to treatment after four years of consistent discomfort in their assigned gender. The onset of their depression began around 13 years old, roughly a year after starting puberty and their first period. Sam reported such dysphoria with their chest growth that there were a few past incidents of self-harm—primarily cuts on their chest. They informed me that they felt largely betrayed by their body and felt no connection or love for it. Sam was once a high achieving and successful student and now their parents can barely get Sam to attend school regularly due to severe anxiety and depression. Sam recently disclosed to therapist that while they still identify as nonbinary, transmasculine, they have a desire to start HRT and eventually pursue top surgery. They don't know how to talk to their parents about this since their parents are already struggling to understand nonbinary gender identities.

Because this is an active time for puberty, adolescence is another primary phase of development where gender dysphoria becomes more apparent. The treatment needs of gender nonconforming children and trans youth are vastly different. Gender nonconforming children are most often very happy once they can achieve feelings of alignment through their gender expression; most of the work is with the family and the parents. On the other hand, trans teenagers navigating puberty are more likely to experience high levels of distress and need more systemic and comprehensive intervention. Trans teens also experience an additional layer of complexity in what they need, which will include invasive and non-invasive interventions to cope with hormonal changes associated with puberty. Relationships also become more complicated at this stage of life. Not only with the changing parental–child relationship, but peer relationships become highly complex and riddled with ever-maturing context and interactions. In addition to nurturing the gender identity and social support from family, peers, and community, trans teens need to develop coping skills and ego strengthening to support their developing self and gender-actualization process.

While treatment approaches with trans teens have similarities with adults, it's important to acknowledge lifespan development. Adolescence is a time of significant identity development, including reflection about what it means to be a gender. For cis people, it's looking into how they want to be a man or woman and how this fits into how they are. For gender diverse folx, this same process is going on, but at the same time they are trying to process the extra stuff that cis people don't have to deal with, such as sorting through internalized stigma, figuring out what gender diversity means, the coming out process, defining transition, and feelings of starting from scratch, while everyone else seems ahead in figuring out who they are. For all adolescents, this stage of development is incredibly significant for the brain as it undergoes rapid and drastic changes surrounding impulse control, cognitive reasoning, emotional processing, abstract and rational thinking, and grasping social constructs and relationships. Distress tolerance is a highly important skill all teenagers would benefit from. It's at the core of treatment modalities for teens.

My process for standard assessment of trans identifying teens is affirming and thorough. It's important to have a concrete process for working with gender diverse minors and informing parents and guardians of this. First, WPATH, DSM-5, and my Gender Dysphoria Assessment are my go-to for diagnostic support. The additional factor in assessment of trans teens is the waiting protocol. There is a general rule that the teen must be in therapy for six months prior to starting HRT. Hormone replacement therapy is not the same as starting hormone blockers. Initiating puberty suppressants is a decision made with the medical provider while the teen and family take time to decide what's next. While some may find this a form of gatekeeping, most find it appropriate. The waiting game is probably the most useful part of the assessment process in working with gender diverse adolescents. While HRT is a generally safe intervention, there are significant and drastically changing aspects of being for a teenager, all thanks to that good ol' rapid brain development. Hormone intervention makes permanent changes, and with anything permanent, it's important to process the impact even if the benefits are drastically better. In these six months, it's important to affirm the gender identity, not challenge its legitimacy. That's not to say there won't be appropriate challenges that promote healthy processing and emotional insight. But by affirming a trans teen you are holding space for them to self-actualize, something trans folx do not have the privilege of experiencing like cis people in daily life. I explain to parents that teenagers are more likely to push back if they attempt to diminish their trans experiences, so why not try affirming it? Not only does this suggestion promote the autonomy of the client but encourages healthy family practices that will expand the space the teen has to actualize.

As a clinician, I find a lot of usefulness within the six-month waiting game. It involves in-depth practical preparation, insight building, emotional processing, organization for support from family and community, and completion of the assessment process. Cis people shouldn't "pass" this assessment, and if they do, they are most definitely the exception to the rule and incredibly rare. Cis people do not really explore gender variance because their gender identity is affirmed by society. There's generally not a strong influence in a cis person's life to question their gender identity. I would challenge that cis people exploring themes of gender are probably seeking to push boundaries for gender expansion rather than experiencing gender dysphoria. There is a core difference in gender dysphoria and exploration. Exploring gender is like having an anchored boat waiting for you while you venture out. Gender dysphoria is like having no boat to return to, there wasn't one in the first place and there's no choice but to swim or drown. The waiting game allows for the cis teens to return to their boats after actualizing the impulse to jump off the boat, and the gender variant teens to understand which direction they want to go next.

A common factor that could contribute to a client pursuing gender identity exploration to conclude they are not trans is level of personality functioning. Social risk taking is higher in those with lower personality functioning due to diminished sense of self. Personality functioning is always something I am assessing, but I will not gatekeep if a client presents symptoms or diagnoses pertaining to lower personality functioning. This is because the symptoms can be impacted by gender dysphoria or can be co-occurring. If a client presents both gender dysphoria and lower personality functioning, I provide a thorough explanation of my assessment and psychoeducation to both parents and client, as all gender therapists should following their assessment. In my experience, most times personality functioning improves with transition, but this isn't a guarantee. It's also important to remember that it's developmentally appropriate for personality functioning to change at this stage of life due to the drastic changes and adjustments occurring in identity, life stage, and interpersonal relationships. Personality functioning is a wavering experience for all humans as we navigate challenges in life and can be an indicator of surviving trauma.

Protective factors for trans teens are very important to understand because this population is high risk. This group is high risk due to the complex intersection of a marginalized identity, mental health impact due to possible unwanted physiological changes with puberty and internalized stigma, adolescence phase of development, and overall powerlessness to control transition needs independently. Adolescence is a time with intense focus on identity development and social relationships, and these two experiences are drastically impacted by gender identity. The most important protective factor in reduction of suicide risk is parental/familial support. Family rejection is directly linked to poor outcomes and suicidality in trans youth.

In a systematic review of the empirical literature on protective factors for gender variant youth, from Johns et al. (2018), 27 factors for well-being were identified through 21 peer-reviewed articles. But only seven of those factors were deemed protective. Factors identified included: self-esteem, parental support, peer support, trusted adult support, school support, teacher support, and social support. It was recognized how these factors are highly relationally based, even self-esteem, since it is common for self-esteem to be influenced by health of relationships. Gender is a social experience, so gender variance can be an especially complicated experience in adolescence.

Since access for HRT and affirming interventions is relatively newer for trans youth, research will take a while to provide more concrete information about the medical and psychological impact of transition. One study suggests early intervention with hormonal suppression significantly improves daily functioning, decreases depressive symptoms, and reduced behavioral issues. This same study showed that 70/70 participants were still using hormonal intervention; participants were ages 12–16 and the study was conducted over eight years (de Vries, Steensma, Doreleijers, & Cohen-Kettenis, 2011). Another study in 2015 supported these findings with 201 participants who were assessed 6 and 12 months after initiating puberty suppression hormones. Results showed significant improvement in both psychological and daily functioning (Costa et al., 2015). We still have time to find out even longer term impact of hormonal intervention, while shorter term studies are showing clinically significant positive impact.

When working with gender diverse children and teens, I take a strong stance in not outing my clients to their parents. If a minor discloses their gender identity to me, I will protect that information to the greatest extent I can. Some clinicians will refrain from documenting this information since parents have rights to records. Minors technically do not have confidentiality; thus, parents have the right to get involved in treatment. Minors do have a right as a client to privacy and a clinician who will do their best within their ability to keep as much information disclosed in sessions private. Outing a client to their parent or guardian without the collaboration and permission is high risk for harm and damage. When working with minors, I address with parents immediately in the first session that I do not out clients and protect as much privacy as possible. Below is a statement from my informed consent that I review with parents.

Minors

If you are under 18 years of age, please be aware that the law may provide your parents the right to examine your treatment records. It is my policy to ask parents to give up this right. If they agree, I will provide them with only general information about our work together, unless I feel that there is high risk that you will harm yourself or someone else. In this case, I will notify them of my concern. I will also provide them with a summary of your treatment when it is complete. Before giving them any information, I will discuss this matter with you, if possible, and do my best to handle any objections you may have about what I am prepared to discuss.

As I specialize in LGBTQ+ populations, it is important to note that I do not "out" my clients to their families. This means that the gender and sexual identity of my clients are private and confidential information that stays between us. There are many ethical and legal considerations regarding the protection of the rights of minors, and as part of my clinical practice, I do not disclose such information.

Conversations with trans youth are an important aspect of their exploration process because it begins to introduce important decision-making skills that support future autonomy. During the process of initiating dialogue about important considerations regarding transition, clinicians should be careful in their approach to subjects. Be sure to inform the client of your intentions. Marginalized groups, including trans folx, have complex traumatic experiences with gatekeeping from trusted services providers. For trans youth, there can be an additional mistrust of adults because for some, adults have been the primary gatekeepers or perpetuators of stigma. To ensure my intention is upfront, I will inform my teen clients that gender actualization takes reflective work and taking the time to explore and process impact of their impending changes. Initiating these discussions is also holding space for teens to anchor in their ideas and feelings about gender identity and transition. Many conversations are similar to those that should be discussed with adults.

Some conversations that need to be had with trans teens during the first 6 months of gender therapy are as follows.

How Do You Need to Be Seen? What Aspects of Your Social/World Interactions Need to Adjust to Affirm Your Identity?

This is the initial exploration of how the teen identifies. It can be within the binary or nonbinary realms of gender identity. Gender actualization looks different for all folx, and exploring affirming needs to support their gender identity is the most important and primary step of gender therapy. This is a time to explore expressive, social, and existential goals of transition. This conversation should also explore what areas of support are in place because youth do not have autonomy to seek their own affirming resources and interventions. Because of the complexity of lack of overall autonomy, assessing what supports are in place and which need to develop is important for overall outcomes. Identifying what areas of life these clients do have control over is also critical for developing resilience. This part of your interview will also inform treatment in what needs to happen within the family to organize and support the child. In Chapter 9 (Appendix 9.1), the Family Support Plan would be helpful for this aspect of interviewing trans youth clients and their support at home.

Understanding of HRT and Its Limits and Benefits. Assessing for Realistic Expectations

While this discussion is also an important one to have with adults, due to stage of development it's even more important to take the time to assess expectations of HRT with teens. Justifiably so, there's a lot of hype surrounding the positive impact of HRT on physiological and psychological alignment. The outcomes of HRT for everyone will be different and unique, and it doesn't instantaneously erase challenges and speed up self-actualization. Starting hormones is essentially the door opening to begin a process of healing and reclaiming and learning to connect to the self; it's still the early stages of actualization. Just as all genders, hormone's impact on the body may not produce all desired effects. It's also not a medication to take the mental toll away. All people, cis and trans, can fall for magical-type thinking, especially when the intense focus on a specific goal (like starting HRT) has been a long journey to reach.

It would be wise to even graze hard conversations, such as if the client changes their mind. This is something therapists also need to be okay with. Assessing for gender dysphoria has been thrust upon us due to stigma in the medical and insurance fields. Gender dysphoria should be treated as a medical one rather than a psychological one. While we have a thorough and clinically informed process of assessing for gender dysphoria, it doesn't mean there won't be folx who either change their course and decisions regarding transition or completely de-transition. De-transition, according to my experience and the experiences of my peers in this niche, is very rare. So rare, that it should be treated as an exception and not the rule. Some teens have stopped hormones while recognizing there are gender diverse experiences, but maybe a certain intervention isn't impacting dysphoria in the way they thought. Humanity is messy, and clients can always change their course or understanding of who they are. So, while gender therapists need to be okay with that fact that they might have a few clients over the course of their careers change direction, we can also explore this with clients in a way that doesn't introduce stigma or doubt. I will ask clients about being okay with the permanent changes and impact of hormones even if they decided to stop one day.

Reproductive Goals

While a trans teen understands they want hormone intervention, not all may fully grasp that this action can permanently impact reproductive goals in the future. Referring back to the information presented in Chapter 4, teenagers have the right to be informed and process these ideas no matter how mature a therapist might find the concept. It's easy to say as a teen "I don't want kids" or "I'll just adopt," and many clinicians will simply accept this answer and move on. But it's very different when someone is thinking about goals surrounding reproduction after 25, and this decision is being made in a completely different stage of life and development for their future self. They will be a completely different person after 25 with different goals and desires in life. This isn't to say a teen doesn't have a say, it's just important to take time to process as much as the client is willing to go. Having this conversation also supports that developing autonomy of adolescents. If trans teens are to pursue changes that are quite serious, they should be given the respect of the informed consent process medically and psychologically; it is teaching processing skills important for their future.

Initiating this chat is not about assuming the teen will change their mind, it's about the teen having an understanding that they may not want kids right now and may continue to not want them in the future—but there's also a possibility that their mind can change because they are a growing person and people do change their minds. It's about the teen understanding this concept concretely while moving forward, not intentioned to gatekeep. Teens still deserve to be informed in their decision making, even while making decisions about their bodies in youth.

Working with Gender Diversity in the School Setting

School-based counselors are placed in such a unique position. These providers serve as a triangular liaison between student (client), family, and school. This makes for some complex mediating. Included at the end of Chapter 7 is a list of resources, several are included for those working in schools (GLSEN is my favorite). The most challenging aspect of working with trans youth surrounds the difficulties in trying to help and affirm a minor while accepting limitations of working with minors without being out or are out without support. School-based counselors should acknowledge that working with gender diversity is an inevitable part of their job (if it hasn't already come up). Youth are in a critical age of identity development and self-actualization, which means many folx are better understanding their gender identity. Puberty is also a major trigger for dysphoria. Because this will be an inevitable aspect of the position, school-based therapists should seek some form of training and consultation to feel comfortable working with gender diversity in the school.

Gender identity is treated just like any other confidential aspect of treatment. If the student is not ready to come out, it's the role of the clinician to hold affirming space as they begin their process of gender actualization. Do not out the child to parents or school staff without appropriate permission. I include in my consent document that I do not out minors to parents due to the risk and harm to the client. If the student is out, the school-based therapist is to advocate for the student (just like any other clients who need special support from the school) and to work with the family. I also encourage school-based providers to affirm the identity no matter what. If a parent asks me not to use their chosen name or pronoun, I inform the parent that I won't be doing that because it's harmful to my client and not best practice. I am quite transparent with schools and parents that I come from an affirming place and will support children as they actualize their gender. A critical difference between my setting and private practice and a school-based provider is the entanglement of several roles. Many school-based providers are affiliated with another community-based agency or practice, work for the school too, and provide services for a minor under the parents. There are a lot of voices and opinions. I would start with the source and work my way through, address the affiliation (practice or agency) about affirming policies and practices, then the school, and this will then translate to parents.

The primary theme in both standard practice and outcomes data is the importance of organizing support—mainly from family. Addressing the family system is as important, if not more important, than the individual work with the client. While the individual work with trans youth can be inspired by personal clinical orientation and some interventions I addressed in previous chapters, working with the families can be intimidating. In Chapter 9, I outline transitioning families and detail each stage. The phases of transitioning families are influenced greatly by grief, but provide the clinician and clients with a concrete concept of what to expect as families tackle transition and its impact on their system.

Reflection Questions for Clinicians

1   What is your reaction to puberty suppressants for prepubescent gender diverse children?
2   What factors do you feel contribute to parental/guardian resistance?
3   How do you want to handle gender diverse minors in your clinical practice? What will your informed approach with families and clients from the beginning, assessment, and treatment look like? Collect your local resources.

References

Costa, R., Dunsford, M., Skagerberg, E., Holt, V., Carmichael, P., & Colizzi, M. (2015). Psychological support, puberty suppression, and psychosocial functioning in adolescents with gender dysphoria. *The Journal of Sexual Medicine*, 12(11), 2206–2214. https://doi.org/10.1111/jsm.13034

de Vries, A. L., Steensma, T. D., Doreleijers, T. A., & Cohen-Kettenis, P. T. (2011). Puberty suppression in adolescents with gender identity disorder: a prospective follow-up study. *The Journal of Sexual Medicine*, 8(8), 2276–2283. https://doi.org/10.1111/j.1743-6109.2010.01943.x

Johns, M. M., Beltran, O., Armstrong, H. L., Jayne, P. E., & Barrios, L. C. (2018). Protective factors among transgender and gender variant youth: a systematic review by socioecological level. *The Journal of Primary Prevention*, 39(3), 263–301. https://doi.org/10.1007/s10935-018-0508-9

Rae, J. R., Gülgöz, S., Durwood, L., DeMeules, M., Lowe, R., Lindquist, G., & Olson, K. R. (2019). Predicting early-childhood gender transitions. *Psychological Science*, 30(5), 669–681.

9 Transitioning Families

Co-authored by Butch Losey, EdD, LPCC-S

I began co-writing an article with Dr. Butch Losey to combine our expertise. He is a highly experienced systemic therapist and I wanted to combine this lens with my experience working with gender diversity to create a clinical framework for working with transitioning families. We are both two very busy therapists who practically completed our article, but never got around to cleaning it up and having it published. I know, I know, I practically face-palmed just typing that last part. Instead, he agreed I could publish our work in this book since this chapter was going to cover everything we wrote anyway. For this reason, there will be times this chapter reads more like a journal publication.

Families experience transition when a member of their family begins their process of gender actualization. Family members of the trans individual undergo their own changes, such as: challenging deep-rooted binary ideas about gender, social attachment and bonding, reflecting about one's own gender identity and what it means existentially, and how the gender binary has affected interactions with our world. Especially for cis persons, the "bubble popping" moment can be incredibly uncomfortable. The family may feel their emotions are less important or a burden to their gender diverse member, and this can hinder or stagnate the family in integrating this new change within the system. Individuals within the family are processing significant and complicated grief emotions that are normal and expected, and this can impact how the family organizes and adapts. If the grief is not processed or accepted, this can create dysfunctional patterns within the family and its relationships. Parents could be responding to feelings of fear, grief, value confliction, and shock that can potentially result in defensive, stonewalling, blaming, or other ineffective reactionary behaviors. Any change a family undergoes causes a ripple effect that the family then must adapt to. Because of the unique personal and systemic experiences associated with integrating a new gender identity, these families are referred to as "transitioning families."

There are two processes occurring for "families in transition": one is a process of the trans person growing into one's authentic gender identity or gender actualization, and another process is the systemic transformation

DOI: 10.4324/9781003001881-10

of the family. The transgender person gender-actualizes by fully expressing their gender identity and relinquishing the distress of attempting to conform to their assigned gender at birth. The rest of the family transitions to experiencing their loved ones in a more authentic way, many times weaving their way through grief and loss. Systemic transformation requires relational changes, along with deep personal change for family members, best achieved in the context of an affirming environment.

There is a multitude of influences on the path to gender actualization. One strong influence is gender socialization, which starts at birth and continues throughout our lives—the cultural expectations of our roles according to our assigned gender. From birth on, perceived boys and girls are treated differently by family members and others in their world. Children learn quickly the cultural expectations of what it means to be boys and girls and women and men. This gender socialization occurs in multiple contexts of interaction in everyday life, including schools, peer groups, and communities, but it is commonly agreed upon that the family is the most important context in which gender behaviors and identities are learned, formed, and enacted (das Dores Guerreiro, Caetano, & Rodrigues, 2014). Family gender socialization starts even before any child is born in the family, through the parents' own development of parental identity.

Parents are assumed to have stable gender identity and begin to develop their parental identity as they move from adolescents to adulthood. Before the birth of their first child, they have some idea of how they will act as a parent, they know their gender preference for their unborn children, what names they like, how many children they would prefer, and all sort of dreams for this unborn child. When parents begin forming these expectations, hopes, and dreams for their unborn child, they are forming a bond to that child grounded in the context of gender. This attachment influences how the parent will relate and interact to their child after the child is born.

In order to create a sense of security and stability, people base many belief systems and values in binary "this or that" terms. Families do this for gender as well; for example, they can define family members as either male or female. Once defined, there are numerous cultural expectations and social norms and rules to follow. In truth, human identities are incredibly complex and can rarely be defined by binary concepts. Gender is fluid and contains deep complexity. Families can lose this sense of stability when one member begins to express and identify with more fluid gender ideas. For someone who gender actualizes, the process can be seen as two concurrent processes: one process of the individual actualizing and the other process of the family transitioning. This is a difficult process because each part of the system must accommodate changes in the other, and since systems naturally resist change, all members of the family can feel at odds with one another.

Ambiguous Loss

When children and adolescents come out as trans, families often experience a profound sense of grief and disorientation. The family members are often confused about their child's emerging identity and changing role in the family. Parental figures must process the loss of their gender-normative dreams and expectations (Wahlig, 2015). The impact is so significant that family members may feel a destruction of gendered expectations for their child's future—the loss of a particular gender context relationship that they shared before the child came out, and a strong challenge to the gendered identity as the mother or father of a son or daughter. All this change overwhelms the transitioning family with complex and radically conflicting emotions. Defining a concrete experience of grief and loss for parents and families of transitioning children and adolescents is particularly uncertain.

How I define ambiguous loss to systems experiencing transition is chaotic confusion surrounding a profound sense of loss. When someone dies, we understand why we are grieving. There are available resources for grieving individuals who are experiencing a loss through death, and there's a lot of representation in our culture to provide people with at least a small sense of what to expect. With death, families typically come together to support one another, there is usually a funeral and memorial service, and families participate in spiritual practices along with other rituals. Families can comfort and be comforted, and through connection with others bring a sense of closure. This is not what transitioning families experience.

Human brains hate vagueness and will keep ruminating and problem solving to find something concrete that makes sense to explain events or circumstances that are unclear. Ambiguous loss is an exhausting experience to understand the concept of feeling like their loved one is dying or has died, but they are still here. Then this triggers mental systems to try and reconcile even more complex feelings including shame, guilt, anxiety, depression, and loss. In addition to these internal processes, systemically the support system of the family typically is not a source of support. Many times, friends, extended family, and community of the family do not know what to say or do to support the transitioning family. Their messages are confusing as some are silent, some are oppositional towards supporting the transitioning individual, and others may provide supportive feedback. Social support is a primary need during grief, so families are often deprived of this and forced to go within the family to process.

Stages of Family Transition

Family Transition is the accommodation and integration of new gender information within a family unit that encourages exploration and expression of a trans person's authentic gender identity. Successful family transition requires members to be flexible and adaptive because gender actualization is a process that occurs over time. Expansive families can regularly adjust to the changing experiences of the trans person's gender-actualization process. Families experience transition when one member of the family comes out and begins to express their gender in ways that challenge the family's binary ideas about gender. The family will most likely respond by experiencing grief emotions that are normal and expected, impacting interactions within the family. If grief is not addressed and integrated into treatment, this can create tension and distance within the family as they will feel distanced by internal and unresolved grief emotions. See Table 9.1 for family stages of transition.

Families that are overwhelmed with grief are more likely to reject family transition and the gender identity of the child or adolescent. These families present in treatment with systemic symptoms of increasing distal and conflictual relationships, perceiving to have innate and unwavering values conflict, lacking a strong understanding of the complex aspects of gender identity, and rejecting efforts of authentic gender expression by the trans person. Transition rejection is internalized by the trans person as rejection of the true self, which increases potential for negative outcomes for the child.

> Family rejection on the basis of sexual orientation and gender identity was the most frequently cited factor contributing to LGBT homelessness. The next most frequently cited reason for LGBT youth homelessness was youth being forced out of their family homes as a result of coming out as lesbian, gay, bisexual, or transgender.
>
> (Durso & Gates, 2012)

Data also support the importance of family acceptance for the overall wellbeing of the trans individual, showing that improved self-esteem and increased resilience to mental health issues are a positive result of family acceptance. Conversely, research shows negative impact of family rejection includes higher rates of suicide attempts, increased risk of substance abuse, and higher instances of depression (Ryan, Russell, Huebner, Diaz, & Sanchez, 2010).

Clinical Example

When Tiffany was three years old she began to question her gender in very simple ways. She was assigned male at birth, and around age 3 and 4 Tiffany began asking her mother questions such as "can I grow up to be a girl?" and "Do I have to grow up to be a man?" Tiffany's father recalled those early years as distressing and confusing, especially when Tiffany made strong statements rejecting her assigned gender, such as "I don't want to live to be a boy." Tiffany's decisive persistence in her female identity continued for months, followed by years.

When Tiffany began school at five the family was soon contacted by concerned school personnel who saw her behavior progressively worsen at school. Several times a week Tiffany would have behavioral outbursts that included hiding under tables and spitting and biting other children. As school concerns increased, Tiffany began counseling.

Tiffany's parents made the decision to allow her to wear feminine "dress-up" clothes at home in an attempt to ease her anxiety; this eventually became a routine for her. As soon as she would come home from school, she would run upstairs and change into princess dresses and refuse to take them off; some nights she would sleep in them. When it was time to go to school, she would express anger, anxiety, and sometimes tantrums because she would have to take off her feminine clothes and replace them with stereotypical male attire.

She later named herself and asked her parents and two older siblings to address her as Tiffany. It was at this time that the two opposing selves, one of assigned gender and one of the actualizing self, were becoming more distinct and separate.

Through grief, doubt, and resistance from extended family members, Tiffany's parents remained supportive of their daughter. Yet, Tiffany's behavior at school continued to deteriorate and she began to refuse to go to school. School mornings for Tiffany became battles to avoid school; she was tearful and unable to be soothed.

After many long discussions, her parents contacted a transgender health clinic to be evaluated, and the family received helpful resources, support, and education about gender nonconforming children. In an attempt to be adaptable to Tiffany's needs, mom and dad made the decision to allow her to begin her gender-actualization process.

Soon after making this decision, dad made the first family appointment. Tiffany came to the initial session confident and outgoing; she was visibly secure in herself. Both parents stated that she seems like a completely different child, a happy and confident child, and that though they feel validated in this observation that they made the right decision, they couldn't help but feel they "abandoned" the child they gave birth to and embraced a new child.

Tiffany's parents were supportive, while open in their struggle with grief, doubts, and resistance from extended family and their community. This process wasn't easy, as the father's parents expressed severe opposition, even attempting to contact the therapist dad hired to influence treatment. Neighbors and schools were less resistant and more in need of guidance from Tiffany's parents, which was especially stressful with mom who struggled with doubt and significant grief emotions. Dad felt like he was trying to balance the pressure from his parents while battling his own grief, explaining he felt very vulnerable and conflicted.

Tiffany went back to her second year of preschool as her authentic self and was welcomed by staff and students. Mom and dad worked hard to allow a smooth transition for her, scheduling meetings with the school, setting boundaries with family, and communicating changes with their community. As mom and dad processed their grief, they found a sense of rightness within the family and a speedy return to a sense of normalcy. Tiffany will continue to express herself in how she identifies, per the recommendation of treating gender nonconforming children, while mom and dad will reconcile the fear of any potential changes to gender identity in the future.

Stage 1: Disbelief

Disbelief has many faces, and its impact is unique for all families. With the influences of denial and rejection, this stage can be the most difficult for parents and families to overcome. Initial assumptions are often reactionary and promptly reject the legitimacy of the gender identity. Disbelief is a defensive action to protect the homeostasis of the family and to remove any danger to ultimately avoid a feeling of ambiguous loss. The grief phase of disbelief can manifest in several behaviors, including doubt, seeking contrary evidence, and avoidance. The perceived threat to homeostasis

Table 9.1 Stages of family transition

Stages of Family Transition	Familial Experience
Disbelief	Doubt
	Shock reaction: avoidance, approach, freeze
	Systemic expansion: resistance/accommodation
Identity Rejection	Criticism
	Invalidation
	Seeking contrary evidence
	Encouraging conformity
	Externalizing blame and control
	Cultural conflict
Conditional Accommodation	Self-preservation
	Superficial tolerance
Detachment	Realization of loss
	Ambiguous loss
	Depression/Grief
Acceptance	Healing the ruptures
	Collaboration
	Seeking supportive resources
Affirming Integration	New normal
	Reattachment
	Family cohesion

within the family during disbelief stage, of the continuing existence of the gender actualizing child in that system, is ever-growing, increasing tension and emotional responses. Externalizing pain is a common reaction to the grief emotions in this stage; transitioning families look outward in search of answers rather than inward. Criticism, fear, and cultural conflict are primary indicators of resistance.

At first disclosure, or when the child "comes out," parents and families experience a devastating blow to a perceived security of their family. This secure picture is one with a clear past, a solid present, and an expectation of the future. The image is based on each individual and their role and place within the family system, and these roles and bonds within the familial relationships have roots in gender. When this security feels threatened, it is a natural response of the system to strike down the perceived threat to the homeostasis of the family. It is an instinctual reaction, a decision made from a shock response, to attack the gender identity that is threatening the system's regulation. The gender identity of the gender actualizing child feels like a large risk to the family because it would mean a loss, thus dysregulating the system. The fight against this invisible threat is confusing and can elicit a variety of emotions and behavioral responses. Emotional reactions are expected as the family navigates grief effectively, including anxiety, sadness, melancholy, anger, irritability, depression, fear, shock, and sorrow. Doubt is a standard response; it's essentially the "due diligence" in analyzing our world. Doubt can become ineffective when its sole purpose is to diminish the perceived threat of the gender actualization of a child. When a family or parental system is organizing against the gender actualizing child's authentic identity, they are resisting change. Doubt is a reaction to shock and can help buffer the intensity of the inevitable emotional reaction due to the sudden exposure to uncontrollable devastation and confusion.

Familial Experience

Though denial serves as a barrier in moving forward, it's a typical response to grief. As mentioned above, grieving is an unavoidable process that every family and parent will experience uniquely after their child comes out. Denial tends to be a reaction to shock and can help buffer the intensity of the inevitable emotional reaction due to the sudden exposure to uncontrollable devastation and confusion. Because of feelings related to ambiguous loss, it can be difficult for individuals within transitioning families to recognize that denial helps them avoid facing grief, because grief would mean there's a significant loss to overcome.

As disbelief serves as a barrier in forward progression, avoidance is a complete halt. Avoidance is the action of delaying the grief process by evading dialogue or personal reflection about embracing the emerging gender identity; it's a sort of "waiting it out" strategy. In order to avoid the complex feelings of ambiguous loss, ignoring progressive action is a standard reaction. Essentially, this is avoiding change and the emotions that follow. Transitioning families and parents may resist connecting to appropriate resources and engaging in affirming discussions with their gender actualizing child, hoping the trans identity is temporary and the "identity crisis" will pass. Accepting grief would mean accepting an imminent and significant loss to overcome.

Additionally, families may deal with this first stage by over-approaching or freezing. Freezing is like avoidance but carries less conscious intention. Avoidance is more often the action of purposefully not engaging, while freezing is more of a collective game of unintentional chicken; who's going to cave and initiate conversation about this first? And the opposite of avoidance is the complete lack thereof. Approaching can be excessive when inspired by disbelief because of the anxiety driving it. Sometimes parents can initiate dialogue about the disclosure with desperation to influence and persuade the child that they are not trans. Resistance is expansive: the stage of resistance can be viewed as a stage of expansion. This is because there are multiple processes at work to apply pressure on the family and when this pressure persists, it leads to multiple accommodations. There can be considerable resistance from family members when one member begins to express gender in a different way. Sometimes this resistance is expressed through statements: "this is just a phase" or "my child is misguided."

It's important to note that examples of each phase of family transition and the co-occurring grief responses are not to be confused with healthy and appropriate assessment or questioning of a transitioning family member. It is normal for individuals to question and digest new information that shocks their world view. When this behavior evolves into a barrier for a transitioning individual to pursue necessary steps towards the quality of life is when this behavior is best challenged. Here are some typical actions or phrases that most align with disbelief:

- Exaggerating wait-time (beyond appropriate) to access important trans resources because "I'm not ready yet."
- Refusing to use or making no progress in using proper pronouns after an extended time has passed. Do not confuse this with attempts and making expected mistakes.
- Attributing this disclosure to social media's influence.

"When I was their age, I had no idea who I was either"
"I don't completely feel like a girl/boy sometimes either"
"How can they possibly understand something like that?"
"It's just a phase"
"This stuff is a trend right now"
"My child has lied before to get attention"
"I was confused at their age"
Tasks of Family

Grief is a normal and necessary reaction to new information that shocks one's world view. It is a healthy and appropriate process for the transitioning family to assess any new changes to the system with due diligence. The frustrating conclusion parents and families must come to in order to move beyond this phase is that the legitimacy of their child's identity can only be expressed by the child themself. There is currently no in-depth formal psychological assessment or test to determine if the gender actualizing child is trans or not; it can only be determined by the child's report. Human identities are gray matter in the brain (including gender identity and sexual identity) and form a deeply personal and unique reflection of who we are; there is no scientific method that can evaluate this. It is important for transitioning families and parents to connect to well-rounded information and educational resources to help navigate the symptoms of disbelief.

Stage 2: Identity Rejection

Identity rejection is the emotional reactionary time that can occur beyond disbelief. Because of the unwavering continuity of the disclosed gender identity, transitioning families and parents begin to fathom a potential for permanence. This perceived threat to homeostasis within the family, this continuing existence of the trans identity, is ever-growing, increasing tension and emotional responses. Externalizing pain is a common reaction to the grief emotions in this stage as transitioning family members look outward in search of answers rather than inward. This stage is best defined by its title; the transitioning family will outright reject the trans identity, which ultimately translates in rejecting the child. This is an attempt to terminate the perceived threat to the sense of security in the family system. Criticism, fear, and cultural conflict are primary symptoms of this resistance.

Family values and culture are sacred; it's the glue that holds the family system together with the expectation that they will be honored and carried out by all members. Parents are the core of the family and children are an extension, meaning the source of culture and values are from the parents. Parents orchestrate and lead the family, and if parents are experiencing conflict between values and the gender actualizing needs of their child, the entire family will feel the impact. In addition to reconciling religious, political, cultural, and worldview beliefs, transitioning families are faced with challenging their own preconceived notions about gender. These ideas about gender begin forming in family of origin and are fostered by social experiences with the world. Assuming that other members of the family identify as cisgender, people born cisgender do not have comparable experiences to a trans person.

The behavioral responses of doubt favor dismissive tactics to invalidate the integrity and legitimacy of the child's reported gender identity. Criticism is an expression of disapproval deriving from a negative connotation of the child's experience of their gender. The spectrum of critical behavior ranges, and is not exclusive to blame, dismissiveness, emotional and/or verbal withdrawal, and potentially harmful challenges, sometimes in the form of scare tactics. Externalizing blame derives from the presumption that the gender actualizing child is misguided or naive. Dismissive tactics and criticism paired with the perception of being out of control can lead parents to make accusations towards media, friend groups, or other outward targets. To regain a sense of control, it is not uncommon for parents and transitioning families to make requests to the child's mental provider, school staff, or counselor to withhold support of the gender actualizing child's identity. At times parents may attempt to influence treatment or assessment with the child's therapist, asking the therapist not to affirm the child's identity, resist any discussion about transition, and to arrange treatment around coping with the gender identity without talk of transition. Parents may ask schoolteachers and other providers to refrain from using chosen name or pronouns, minimizing child's exposure to affirming resources.

Consistent with appropriate parental responsibility, healthy challenges are a normal and expected aspect of effective parenting. When transitioning families are in the resistance phase, challenges can be impacted by grief and manifest as dismissive behavior, scare tactics, and emotional withdrawal. Challenges are a method of testing the gender actualizing child and their determination to self-actualize. If the child can pass these tests and prove a sense of consistence and persistence, parents hope a sense of rightness will guide next steps. The problem is, there's often an underlying anticipation, a doubt in the child's identity, and when the child doesn't budge, the test escalates. Dismissiveness is an ongoing invalidation of the legitimacy of the child's report, diminishing child's needs and experiences. Transitioning families may reduce contact, communication, or connection with the child which can feel like shunning. The myth that there is choice in gender identity is incredibly destructive, and scare tactics are an expression of catastrophic inevitable outcomes if the child "chooses" to self-actualize.

An automatic response in all parents is to guard the safety of their child, because they know all too well of the overt negative and oppressive reactions of society to minority and nonconforming groups of people. Many times, parents in their phases of grief are responding to a "conformity equates safety" perspective. As the risk to safety becomes greater, resistance in transitioning families can rise in opposition to meet it. The balance of being a supporter and protector is a difficult task and dealing with an identity that is not accepted by society can trigger an imbalance. Fear responses of transitioning family members are projections of personal fears for the gender actualizing child. Because conformity is safety, transitioning families can mistake that oppressing the gender identity will keep the child safe, protecting them from an irreversible mistake. While the intention is not to cause harm, methods used to challenge the gender actualizing child can manifest into scare tactics that deeply wound the child. This technique can be conscious or unconscious, testing the confidence of child's expressed gender identity. Adults are all too aware of the hardships nonconforming people and minority groups endure in our current society, and it can be instinctual to pressure conformity in children and teens; yet, it is the opposite of safety for trans and LGBTQ+ individuals.

These fixed perceptions are dangerous because families can always muster misplaced evidence to justify their ideas about the legitimacy of their child's report. I often hear numerous stories from families to discount the honesty or truth of the trans individual. Not only does this include perceiving the child is experiencing a social trend or phase, but parents will draw conclusions based on their personal shenanigans and identity confusion recalled from their own adolescent experience. The frustrating conclusion parents and families must accept in order to move beyond this phase is that the legitimacy of their child's identity can only be expressed by the child themself. There is currently no in-depth formal psychological assessment or test to determine if your kid is really trans or not; it can only be determined by the child's report. Our identities are gray matter in our brains (including gender identity and sexual identity) and form a deeply personal and unique reflection of who we are; there is no scientific method that can evaluate this.

Some examples of this stage include:

- Intimidating child by sharing negative consequences they will endure for being who they are, such as bullying and lack of social acceptance, putdowns, and absolutes.

  "How will you ever find love?"
  "Life is going to be so much harder for you"
  "You're going to be bullied so badly."
  "People are so cruel; you're going to have such a hard life."
  "You're going to hell."
  "This won't make you happy."

- Emotionally withdrawing or shutting child out can be done out of anger, hurt, or punishment.
- Attributing the identity to another mental health issue or personal need that can't be "fixed" with transition, and blaming external sources such as the internet, social trends, or social support that affirms child.
- Using "never" statements.

  "Your dad will never accept this"
  Tasks of Family

Transitioning families must accept this challenge to their world view and perceptions about gender—to open to multi-perspective approach while educating self and engaging with child. Much like the previous stage, it is important for the transitioning family to identify normal grief reaction and feel empowered to do the work. Families can seek unbiased information, consultation with professionals who work with trans people, and process with trusted individuals within their social circle that are safe and appropriate for this type of situation. Parents can vulnerably share their process of trying to move into a supportive position with their actualizing child. This could empower the child to better understand the behaviors and emotions being observed rather than drawing their own conclusions that might be distorted and harmful. Some transitioning families may decide to try consulting with a therapist or medical provider at this stage.

Stage 3: Conditional Accommodation

Conditional accommodations are made as the transitioning family takes a step forward towards acknowledging the permanency in the child teen's gender identity. This is essentially the start of "negotiations," the beginning steps towards the adaptation within the family system. While arrangements are forming and this indicates positive progression, families still show in the types of compromises that are agreed upon. There are contextual obligations set in place for the gender actualizing child that tend to prioritize comfort of the transitioning family members. The negotiations vary in nature between context rejection and circumstantial acceptance. The rejection of the gender actualizing child's gender identity may change depending on the environment. An example might be the gender identity is tolerated at home while at school the child is expected to keep their gender a secret. Acceptance may fluctuate depending on the bargain and is often based on placating the trans person enough to keep control of disclosure and transition. This doesn't necessarily have bad intention behind it because parents naturally seek control in big situations involving their child to try and maintain safety and boundaries.

Self-Preservation

A common grief response is a heightened focus on personal needs. Self-preservation feels like a necessity to survive the crisis or threat. While the transitioning family navigates complex grief experiences, they become clouded in their ability to fully nurture needs of gender actualizing child. The behavioral response manifests in prioritizing the needs of self and family over the gender actualizing child, and this poses a risk because it can delay the child from accessing needed resources or interventions. The most common response of a transitioning family member is "I'm not ready," and this ultimately postpones needed progression to alleviate distress of the child. This poses a significant risk to the emotional and physical safety of the gender actualizing person as it strips away power and oppresses the emergence of their true and authentic self.

Superficial Tolerance

Superficial tolerance is the practice of giving shallow acceptance of the child's gender identity by allowing limited and controlled space for the child to express themselves. As negotiations are underway, rules are established to hide the child's gender identity within certain contexts for needs of the transitioning family. While there are conditions that request suppression, permissions are also granted to entice obedience from the gender actualizing child. Superficial accommodations for gender-actualization needs are made for the purpose of placating the child, while also setting conditions for child to access them. Tolerating the gender identity in order to control the process of gender actualization is a tactic to restrict progress the family may not be ready to manage. This may indicate the transitioning family has not yet established a "united front" and fear external confrontation from external systems, including extended family, community, and peers. A united front is a way to shield and protect the family from outside influences that may impact the adaptation process of the family.

Examples of Conditional Acceptance:

- Parent offering a change they can provide (while feeling initially uncomfortable, in reality it's within their comfort level enough to offer it) while expecting compliance from child or teen for a set of conditions in accepting the accommodation from parent.
- Parent continually expressing they are not ready for progress to justify not progressing, and instead offering small ways to affirm child/teen and expecting it to be enough.

    "I will buy you the binder if you wear girl clothes to family Christmas this year."
    "I will use your name and pronouns at home, but not when we are outside of this house."

Tasks of Family

As the family continues to process the grief emotions eliciting contextual rejecting behaviors, it is important for families to recognize contributing factors and triggers to their circumstantial discomfort with the child's authentic gender expression. A therapeutic setting would benefit the transitioning family to formulate a family support plan (see Appendix 9.1) that includes more balanced preparation to organize around gender actualizing child's process. This setting would also provide opportunity to learn and implement effective communication skills to increase vulnerability and emotion-centered dialogue. Consistent communication within the family is necessary as negotiations are an ongoing aspect of transition in the family. During negotiations, the transitioning family is expected to increase the gender actualizing child's needs within agreements to challenge self-preservation impulse.

Stage 4: Detachment

In order to establish a relationship with the "new child," a form of detachment is necessary for re-bonding and connection. Even though the gender actualizing child has not died, the transitioning family is experiencing a deep sense of loss that can feel like a death occurred. Since gender is a social construct that influences daily interactions and experiences with society and our world, it directly impacts the formation of relationships and attachments between people. Now that the gender actualizing child is pursuing authenticity, it challenges the family to sever the old bond in order to transform the attachment and re-establish a new bond. Essentially, the entire context of the relationship is changing, which calls for complete reorganization. This phase of detachment signifies a turning point for the transitioning family because it's the start of the necessary adaptation process for the family. Grieving is most apparent in this phase of the transitioning family. Families are navigating the realization of the loss and grasping the confusing experiences of ambiguous loss. Depression emerges from the heart of the grief and indicates the family member is vulnerable and open. This stage often exhibits a decreased presence of defense mechanisms acting as a barrier toward acceptance.

Realization of Loss and Ambiguous Loss

Realization of the loss is the understanding that this experience in familial transition signifies a loss and there's nothing left to do except coming to terms with and accepting these feelings. Ambiguous loss is the confusion about the type of loss that is occurring. It's feeling the full impact of grief while not having concrete answers to grasp on to. This ambiguity leaves a layer of confusion and sometimes this uncertainty can create resentment towards the personified gender identity. This appears as a dislike for the child's persona of the actualized gender, as if they're a different person taking the place of the perceived lost child. This internal disorientation sheds light on the heavy influence social constructs have had in the attachment and relational development between parent and child.

In some ways, the gender actualizing child will experience significant personal changes, while there will also be many core aspects of self that will remain constant. The unknown about what's on the other side of transition and self-actualization is a primary trigger of ambiguous loss. The gender actualizing child is still existing, they haven't died, and their being is merely changing a context, the context of gender. Gender actualization is an existential journey for the transitioning person, and this leads to inevitable changes to characteristics and personality; these other forms of development are inevitable due to such a growth and manifestation of authenticity. Transitioning families also grapple with an internal dilemma that by embracing this new identity, they are ultimately abandoning the child that was.

Depression\Grief

Depression is the most recognized symptom of grief that results from embracing the loss and the complexity of feelings that come with that. There is a concrete reality and understanding that the gender identity is permanent and there's nothing left to do but accept this new truth. Sufferers are burdened with a sense of frequent melancholy accompanied by inconsistent lows of despair and devastation. Eventually as grief runs its course, there is more predictability and stability of mood, and the presence of depressive days decrease. Depression marks the start of accepting the reality beyond conditional acceptance. It's the sobering moment that there is no going back and it's time to accept the real feelings of loss; this often resembles processing a death. In order to begin re-bonding, familial reorganizing, and welcoming new changes, the transitioning family has to let go to of the perceptions and dreams held from the past. The transitioning family is encouraged to embrace the vulnerability and release feelings of guilt.

Standard examples in this stage:

- Stages and symptoms of grief.
- Depression and possibly hopelessness.
- Powerlessness. It can feel like you can't stop an avoidable loss, even though the loss is not avoidable.
- Feeling lost.
- Many parents feel like they are abandoning their child to embrace a new one.
- Feeling as if someone has died, but they haven't—causing confusion and shame.

Tasks of Family

Since grief is largely present during this phase of familial transition, processing grief and pain are critical and at the forefront. Much like a death, it is necessary to let go of and transform the dreams that began prior to the child's birth. With any loss, there is a time to say goodbye and accepting the reality of the loss. As the family navigates the complexities of ambiguous loss and depression, it is important to continue emotional and vulnerable dialogue. By keeping feelings of grief withheld, the gender actualizing child can misread events within the family and will then internalize guilt and shame. Grief needs to be normalized for the entire family, including the gender actualizing child, in order to unite rather than distance the family in their adjustment process. When the family can embrace the change and its normal feelings together, it's pretty typical for the storm to pass more quickly. If the family is struggling to engage in healing and vulnerable discussions together, meeting with a gender affirming family therapist could help this process. Sometimes it can be helpful for parents or other grieving family members to process raw thoughts and feelings in private with a therapist before feeling ready to move onto the next steps.

Stage 5: Acceptance

The stage of acceptance begins a time of movement for the transitioning family. The early stages were phases of resistance, followed by embracing loss and accepting change is coming, and finally the family moves towards re-organization and integrating change within the system. It is not uncommon for ruptures to occur when the family system has to adapt to new large changes. During this phase of acceptance, it's important for the transitioning family members to take responsibility and work to heal wounds that have occurred as a result of going through the messy process of transition. The family then works on creating a more united front and undergoes talks about how to unite as a family in support of the gender actualizing child as they transition.

Healing the Ruptures

The roller coaster ride of grief is not an easy ride for anyone who's involved. The experience causes some bumps and bruises along the way, and it's time to tend to the wounds. During the course of the transition within the family, unpredictable and impulsive emotions take a lead, prompting conflict, hurt feelings, and relationship ruptures. Ruptures are events in a relationship that triggers a rift or emotional separation. Ruptures create a guarded emotional and physical distance as a result of negative interactions. When a relationship lacks vulnerability, it lacks trust. Healing these wounds is determined by the process of rebuilding vulnerability and trust. Healing communication is about attentiveness to one another's experiences and taking accountability and responsibility for your part in the ruptures. This means discussing the impact grieving behaviors had on the one-on-one relationships, the family, and the gender actualizing child, and validating the multi-perspectives. Repairing ruptures also involve negotiation of relational needs and practicing consistency in new relationship agreements.

Seek Supportive Resources and Collaboration

As the family is no longer perceiving the trans identity as a threat, there is more willingness to connect with resources that are in support of the gender actualizing child. The family is ready to engage in local resources and connections in the area: support groups, mental health counseling, family counseling, couple's counselor, gender therapy, medical consultations, and LGBTQ+ or Trans centers. The transitioning family is in a place of mobility, ready to back up the actualizing child on their path. Seeking supportive resources is a sign that the family is no longer aligning in opposition against the trans identity and is instead coming to accept the new normal.

Collaboration during the acceptance phase indicates that conditional accommodations are expiring. Instead of biased and linear agreements, the family is negotiating systemically with the needs of the gender actualizing child. At this stage, the family is aligning with the comfort and needs of the gender actualizing child and recognizing the permanence. The family is now understanding that with permanence of the trans identity, conditional tolerance and superficial accommodations are no longer appropriate or relevant. The collaborative process includes consistent engagement in supportive resources, vulnerable and healing communication, and circular and inclusive agreements for family adaptation.

Tasks of the Family

At this stage, the goal is consistency of positive changes. The family needs consistency in follow-up with supportive resources, communication, and accommodation. For the lingering grieving process, this may also be a time of finding ways to stay connected to the "lost person" while moving on in relationship with the "new person." It is expected that at this stage the transitioning family is encouraging authentic gender expression and actively challenging binary perspectives of gender.

Stage 6: Affirming Integration

The sixth and final stage for transitioning families re-establishes a sense of homeostasis and security within the system. Affirming integration is a collaborative rhythm where unconditional positive regard reigns and the environment is safe for gender actualization to develop. This phase is considered the "post transition" phase for families and normalcy has a new context and meaning for the family culture. As the gender actualizing child defines and implements their transition, the family members now organize and adopt an affirming stance to integrate and support gender development.

Family Cohesion

Family cohesion is established when the family is functioning as a team to support and affirm the gender actualizing child. The family is now aligning against negative external factors rather than the transitioning child. When a family is actively practicing this cohesion, it acts as a protective shield against potentially harmful influences from the community, extended family and relationships, and the world. The united front resists outward vulnerability to repel persuasion from the mesosystem and macrosystem in order to protect the new homeostasis and regained functioning within the family system. This practice is necessary to maintain strength in the process achieved by the transitioning family.

Reattachment

Reattachment is the process of establishing the new bond with the gender actualizing child. This change comes with the understanding that the gender actualizing child is not necessarily a "new child," but the "old child" within a new context. Reattachment can increase a sense of closeness and emotional intimacy as transitioning family members have a chance to bond to the authentic identity. As the relational ruptures continue to heal, the wounds are replaced with strengthening trust and vulnerability, and a new and more authentic relationship can begin existing between the gender actualizing child and the family.

New Normal

The new normal is now the gender actualizing child feels affirmed within the familial system and the family has regained homeostasis once again. The family and child anticipate future milestones and are prepared to manage them as a team. The family culture now includes inclusivity of gender and works hard to accommodate needs of affirming gender actualization. There may be times where a family member revisits another phase of transition, as there are many more developmental milestones that the gender actualizing child and family will experience. The new normal grants the gift of knowledge and experience, skills that the family will use to navigate future developments.

Tasks of the Family

As the family has moved into a functioning state of homeostasis, the task of the family is to refocus on relationship building and uniting as a family under the new culture. The family is to establish an authentic and affirming relationship with gender actualizing child and engage in a new bonding process. As the family establishes their united front, family members now adopt roles as liaisons and advocates to protect the new homeostasis achieved within the system. The transitioning family can expect a potential revisit to previous stages of transition as gender developmental milestones can trigger grief or other deep emotions.

Brill and Pepper (2008), in *The Transgender Child: A Handbook for Families and Professionals*, suggest that the parents who ascribe to the vow of parental acceptance promise to follow eight principles:

1   Speak positively about my child to them and to others about them.
2   Take an active stance against discrimination.
3   Make positive comments about gender diversity.

4   Work with schools and other institutions to make these places safer for gender variant, transgender, and all children.
5   Find gender variant friends and create our own community.
6   Express admiration for my child's identity and expression, whatever direction that may take.
7   Volunteer for gender organizations to learn more and to further the understanding of others.
8   Believe my child can have a happy future.

Adult Trans Children

These stages of the transitioning family can be applied to families of adult trans children, while there are also additional considerations. The primary difference is level of influence and power of parents and family over the transitioning adult. Because of this, there can be an increased intensity of reaction of parents and family members in response to feelings of powerlessness and not feeling heard. This autonomy of the transitioning adult can also result in increased boundaries to protect their transition process. This push and pull from family and the gender actualizing adult can result in significant ruptures to the relationship.

It is normal and healthy for adult children to seek and create personal independence to establish the sense of self beyond their family of origin. This is a difficult developmental stage for parents and guardians of origin as it's a change in relationship and parental identity. Parents and guardians are accustomed to being a primary voice in major decisions for their children until adulthood, and it's a difficult transition for children to enter adulthood. When an adult child has come out and made the decision to pursue gender authenticity, this triggers a huge sense of powerlessness, and sometimes a panic, because parents and guardians have adopted the strong duty of protecting their children, which means they have a say in what happens. When parents and guardians do not respond in a supportive manner, or the adult child anticipates resistance, it's a common practice to implement boundaries and leave the family out of their next steps. While this can be a very healthy and safe move for the transitioning person, this can also result in a large trust rupture between family and adult child, another wound to be healed as the family transitions. This is not to say it's the obligation of the transitioning adult child to include the family in this process, because it's not. The emotional and physical safety of the trans person is the most important priority. When speaking to the familial impact, there are many opportunities for relationship wounds and negative interactions.

Because of the sense of powerlessness, it is not uncommon for parents, guardians, or family members of the transitioning adult child to contact care providers supporting transition. I have received long emails, voicemails, and even letters through the mail from parents who know their child is seeing me with intent to transition. Often these letters come from a caring and fearful place, while there is also intent to influence the assessment and treatment process. These parents are serious and sometimes ruthless about their roles as protectors for their children, adult or minor, and it's important to maintain that positive connotation of parents when doing this work. In these times, the clinician also needs to maintain strict boundaries and clinical professionalism by informing client of the contact attempt, and minimally engaging with the family member while not disclosing the adult child's participation in treatment. I typically give a referral to my client to provide to family members struggling with confusion, grief, or relationship rupture.

Recommendations for Therapists

The primary recommendation for therapists when working with transitioning families is to maintain a strong unwavering stance in both supporting the trans child's gender identity unconditionally and holding a positive connotation of the transitioning family. Holding strong ground in both courts simultaneously can get rocky at times, but this consistency is important to model for the entire family. Because research indicates that transgender youth with more accepting and supportive parents may have better mental and physical health outcomes, interventions that increase parental understanding and acceptance are supported. Mental health professionals would benefit from strengthening skills surrounding parental coaching, facilitating high conflict dialogue, and interventions to aid in decision making. Therapists will encounter complex grief, sometimes hostility as a result of resistance, negotiations within family work, and roles as affirming educators. Clinicians should prioritize moving the family towards acceptance and affirming integration as family support is a primary indicator of positive outcomes for trans youth. Family rejection is the primary risk factor for negative outcomes.

Reflection Questions for Clinicians

1 Imagine someone you love came out as trans and is starting transition. Really sit with this scenario and recognize your reactions and emotions.
2 How do you notice the stages of grief appear in the stages of transitioning families?
3 How can you use the information from this chapter in working with transitioning families? How would you present them with this information?

Appendix 9.1

Family Support Plan

Family Support Plan

Client's Name:_____   Date: _____

Client's Identified Gender:_____   Client Age: _____

Client Pronoun(s): _____

Diagnosis (if applicable): _____

FAMILY
Immediate/Primary Family,   **Supportive of Client's Transition?**
list age and if in household   *Yes, No, In Progress*

1.

2.

3.

4.

5.

6.

7.

8.

Additional Factors to be Considered Regarding Family's Involvement in Client's Transition:

What Rules are in Place for Disclosure?

Immediate Family or Friends:

Extended Family or Friends:

School and/or Work:

Peers:

Community:

Additional Considerations Regarding Disclosure:

Who are the client's most significant supports?
1.
2.
3.
4.
5.

What supportive resources are in place for the client and/or family?

What are the current needs of the family to increase support and understanding?
What are the current goals and/or needs of family at this time?

TRANSITION

Who is Client "Out" to?:   **Who is Client not "Out" to?:**

What is the current timeline in place for transition? This includes coming out, mapping what transition looks like, social goals, physical intervention goals (if applicable), and other goals related to integrating gender identity into everyday life (list current plans/ideas below):

Is medical intervention indicated?   Request for letter/collaboration?
YES or NO   YES or NO

What are the most difficult hurdles anticipated during transition? What support does client need to overcome obstacles?

CLIENT GOALS

Level of family involvement needed in treatment:
MINIMAL   LOW   MODERATE   HIGH   EXTREME

How would you rate current progress of family in affirming and integrating
gender identity?
NONE < 0   1   2   3   4   5   6   7   8   9   10   > EXCELLENT

In the client's perspective, what can family do to continue progress? What does
client need to feel supported?

References

Brill, S. & Pepper, R. (2008). *The transgender child: a handbook for families and professionals*. San Francisco, CA: Cleis Press Inc.

das Dores Guerreiro, M., Caetano, A. & Rodrigues, E. (2014). Gendered family lives through the eyes of young people: diversity, permanence and change of gender representations in Portugal. *Gender and Education*, 26 (N1), 35–51, http://dx.doi.org/10.1080/09540253.2013.875130.

Durso, L. E., & Gates, G. J. (2012). *Serving our youth: findings from a national survey of service providers working with lesbian, gay, bisexual, and transgender youth who are homeless or at risk of becoming homeless*. Los Angeles: The Williams Institute with True Colors Fund and The Palette Fund.

Ryan, C., Russell, S. T., Huebner, D., Diaz, R., & Sanchez, J. (2010). Family acceptance in adolescence and the health of LGBT young adults. *Journal of Child and Adolescent Nursing*, 23(4), 205–213.

Wahlig, J. L. (2015). Losing the child they thought they had: therapeutic suggestions for an ambiguous loss perspective with parents of a transgender child. *Journal of GLBT Family Studies*, 11, 305–326.

10 Transitioning Couples

Working with transitioning couples can be incredibly challenging because you're working with two unwavering identities: core aspects of self that are negotiated differently than the conventional sense associated with couple's therapy. Both identities are equally valid, and sometimes the couple can achieve integration and balance, while other times the couple is not able to accomplish this task. It comes down to the ability of the transitioning partner and non-transitioning partner to navigate a completely new relationship. This dynamic can be difficult to direct because of many needs both partners bring to the table. The transitioning partner has needs to transition authentically and feel supported and loved, and the non-transitioning partner needs to process ambiguous loss and grief emotions, while trying to navigate whether they want to continue with the relationship. Both needs are equally important and valid within the relationship, and at times they will combat with one another. The role of the therapist is to facilitate attentive support for both individuals in the relationship while aiding the couple in completely renegotiating the terms and groundwork of their relationship. This chapter will spend most attention to the situation of disclosure of trans identity after the committed long-term relationship was previously established. This chapter is also more geared towards a cis person with a trans person relationship dynamic but can be applicable to a multitude of differing scenarios.

I use the term "transitioning couple" because I see both people within the couple transitioning. Referring to transition, the partner who is not experiencing gender identity transitioning is still experiencing existential transition as they attempt to navigate complex feelings and ideas that challenge core aspects of self and identity. So even though I see both persons within the couple as transitioning because I see it as a process of transformation, I will reserve the term "transitioning partner" for the gender actualizing and trans spouse. To avoid confusion in this chapter, I will label the non-trans partner as the "non-transitioning": the partner who is not transitioning within the context of being trans. This dynamic I've set up of an assumed monogamous cis and trans partner (who started out as a stereotypical straight dynamic prior to transition) is being used to assist my examples and highlight opposing experiences.

DOI: 10.4324/9781003001881-11

Gender is a primary factor in how we attach to people; it influences how we interact and connect with others and how we perceive and experience someone. When a trans individual comes to terms with their identity while in a relationship with someone, this can devastate their partner because the partner fell in love with the person presented at the start of the relationship—a version of the transitioning partner that had aspects of authenticity but under a different context, a veil over it. I explain to my transitioning couples that the transitioning partner is changing their context. This sounds simple enough, but if you take a second to think on this, a change in context is a complete metamorphosis that impacts every facet of the individual, and thus the relationship. Coming from a systemic perspective of recognizing the power of influence and individual can have on their relationship, a change in context of a spouse or partner changes the entire relational context. This is traumatizing to the relationship because it's a change that hits the foundation of the "relationship house."

No matter what the relationship dynamics are, any drastic disclosure or event that changes the core context and foundation of the relationship will cause a complete demolition of the initial relationship house. I use the image of the relationship house due to how clear the similarities are. You have a foundation, and the structure you build as the house represents relationship dynamics; its boundaries (walls), transparency and openness (windows or layout), strength and resilience, its quirks and character, its size and location, all of these things can be metaphors for the relationship. When the event or disclosure occurs, the relationship house has to be rebuilt to better exemplify the new relationship that has grown and changed. The couple can typically draw from the same foundation; there might need to be some repairs. The couple can also use aspects of the previous house in the rebuilding process, but ultimately the relationship needs to reconstruct.

When a couple initially starts therapy after disclosure of gender identity, the couple may or may not be in crisis. If they are in crisis, stabilization is indicated prior to addressing the entirety of the relationship. If the couple is not presenting current crisis, they remain in the same phase of addressing the impact. The phases I am referring to are listed later in this chapter. For now, I want to highlight the differing and conflicting experiences both the transitioning and non-transitioning significant others are experiencing. This is important not only for the therapist's conceptualization, but for educating and normalizing the couple in early treatment. Taking time to address both perspectives within treatment is critical for aligning the couple together against their obstacles.

Non-Transitioning Spouse/Significant Other

First, the non-transitioning partner could be in crisis, especially if they were completely uninformed about their partner's gender identity from the get-go. This means stability needs to be achieved first in order to continue the work. For the non-transitioning partner, the wave of shock can induce trauma-responses as this information is not erasable; there is absolutely no going back after this information is learned. It presents a significant threat not only to the relationship, but to the non-transitioning partner's perception of the entire narrative and history of the relationship. This stage looks very similar to an infidelity case in the initial phase of infidelity treatment. This means the transitioning partner's role is to be consistent, open, transparent, accessible, nurturing, and supportive of the non-transitioning partner. This also means the non-transitioning partner does not have permission to use their partner as a punching bag; it is their responsibility to communicate feelings effectively, manage ineffective outbursts of emotion, and resist avoidance. Once this partner achieves stability after crisis, then it will be time to process grief associated with the loss of the partner they fell in love with.

Ambiguous loss, as mentioned in Chapter 9, is a grief reaction with an added element of confusion. This concept with transitioning couples is identical to transitioning families. With typical grief, most of us think of a death, and most times people have a concrete understanding of why they are experiencing certain emotions, memories, or thoughts. With ambiguous loss, you have all the symptoms of grief, but in this case, there is often a lack of clarity or haziness on why certain experiences are occurring. *My wife/husband is still alive, but why do I feel like they are dying?* Grief in this scenario is incredibly important because it allows the person to undergo the process of letting go so that they can establish a new bond with the transitioning individual, a new relationship with a different meaning. If the relationship had gendered roles, even the tiniest details in the daily dynamics and interaction are changing.

If the non-transitioning partner is straight and cisgender, it can be assumed that this person has most likely not experienced a significant challenge to their sexuality. In a world that accommodates cis and straight people, it's unlikely this partner has had an earth-shattering event that caused a hard look at sexual identity. I often noticed the instinctive reaction from the non-transitioning spouse is flight, stating the relationship simply cannot work now that their significant other isn't the gender they thought they were anymore. This could absolutely be true, and it's a completely valid reason the relationship may end. The sexuality of the non-transitioning partner is just as valid as the gender identity of their transitioning partner. This can be a confusing time because a process of self-actualization surrounding sexuality through attraction and companionship begins for the non-transitioning person. I often encourage the couple that not making a decision right now, out of a reaction, is actually making a decision. This helped with the anxiety surrounding the ambiguity of the relationship and challenge the pressure of feeling obligated to make a decision immediately. The non-transitioning significant other needs time to sit and process. They also need to see the identity of their transitioning partner emerge to gauge if attraction is there for this new person. This is not just a physical attraction I'm referring to, but an emotional one. The authentic identity of the transitioning person, while familiar and ever present for the trans person, has not been revealed to the non-transitioning partner. There is emotional attraction that needs to be explored. Sexuality is fluid for most people, even binary sexualities on the gay and straight spectrums. Sometimes this is enough for the relationship to continue and other times the non-transitioning spouse finds their sexuality doesn't align with the transition. There is also a potential for shame, guilt, and grief on the non-transitioning person's part because of the lack of attraction to the changing person that is important to explore.

Transitioning Spouse/Significant Other

The unique experiences the transitioning partner is typically processing soon after disclosure or coming out are: guilt for not coming out sooner, shame that is triggered by internalized stigma, anxiety about being left, need for affirming support for gender identity, and the additional complexities of self-actualization. Guilt for not coming out sooner is not only a personal reaction, but the transitioning person is also on the receiving end of the grief and shock reaction from their significant other that is often rooted in anger for the lack of disclosure. It's important to take the time to explain to the couple that the transitioning individual rarely, if ever, intends to purposely lie about their gender identity and somehow trick someone to commit to them so they can finally come out. This is a very harmful narrative that perpetuates a lot of societal stigma around the perceived trickery of trans people. Trans folx are just trying to live their lives the best they can with a very limited toolbox they have been given. Society essentially instills stigma around the legitimacy of trans people and how loveable they are. A common occurrence I have seen in my clinical work is folx will fall in love, and all of the sudden, this will finally be "good enough" to where that desire to pursue their authentic gender will finally disappear because falling in love and following that fantasy of a normal life will silence the voice. This is because trans folx are often bombarded with messages that something is wrong with them, and if there's this sense of rightness or normalcy, or if someone loves them in the way they need to be loved, that need to transition won't be so intense and maybe manageable—the "I could be happy with this" bargain. Unfortunately, as time passes, that need for gender actualization doesn't go anywhere because it's an unwavering aspect of the human identity. It might get quieter at points in one's life, but it will always get loud again until the need is fulfilled. The coping skill of distracting oneself with a phase of life or exciting new chapter is a very normal go-to for trans folx in an attempt to avoid addressing their gender identity—the endless pursuit of happiness. Not to say these behaviors don't bring true results, there can be happiness in these pursuits which is why it's the automatic behavior; there's a reward and a feeling of progress.

When a trans individual who isn't out falls in love and doesn't disclose it, many times there is a much deeper story that is rarely given credit or acknowledgment. Marginalized groups of people are only trying to navigate a world with tools they were given by their family and society. Trans people grow up with the narrative that they are unlovable and that if they just found the right things to make them happy, they wouldn't want to transition anymore. So, the hope within the relationship is often times that there will be so much love and happiness, that they will never transition. I have had many clients go back into the closet and regress, ending therapy stating they don't plan to transition because they want to pursue this "easier" path. And as time passes it becomes more impossible each day to fathom coming out to this loved one. Sometimes it can go years, decades. Other times maybe months. Then, when it is finally disclosed or found out (sometimes clues are left intentionally to be caught), it feels like a whole mess that felt like spiraled over time. Communicating this to the couple from the beginning is important for multi-perspective taking and destigmatizing the narrative of deception when intention wasn't initially there. It's also important to express that while intention for harm wasn't there, it's healing for the non-transitioning partner to receive an acknowledgment of a decision to withhold information, which violates most commitment contracts of relationships.

In addition to the guilt, internalized stigma rears its ugly head when disclosure happens in the relationship. Coming out takes a huge level of vulnerability, and coming out within a committed relationship with a loved one brings up the fears of abandonment and the dark reminders of what society has told one to feel about being trans. The internal commentary of being unworthy and unlovable is often playing on repeat. If the trans person had a traumatic experience coming out to family, then being retriggered is a high risk. During this vulnerable time of coming out to a spouse or significant other in a committed relationship, there is high risk of a lot of personal mental health regression due to all the potential triggers that can happen during this process. The relationship is also at a vulnerable time which naturally increases risk of dissolution of the partnership. And this process is going to be sloppy which makes it even riskier because both individuals are having high-intensity emotions driving interactions. All of this increases anxiety and depressive thoughts related to being left and questioning the longevity of the relationship.

In couples therapy, the transitioning person will not get the depth of therapeutic support for their actualization process. This can be frustrating, especially if this partner hasn't sought or had individual therapy to support transition or gender actualization. Couples therapists all have conflicting ideas about how couples and individual therapy should happen, some support individual and couples therapy occurring in tandem and others do not support this. The reason some do not support in tandem work, or are just very cautious with it, is the individual therapy can impact the couples therapy process that negatively impacts progress. Or there are just too many voices at one time and the therapies end up working against each other. Only when I see significant individual needs do I support individual and couples therapy working at the same time. When working with transiting couples, I do strongly support individual gender therapy for the transitioning person, so they have a place to process and actualize their gender. This way, the couples sessions don't distract from the relationship to the individual needs of the transitioning partner. This doesn't mean gender actualization isn't discussed in sessions, it is quite often—as is the grief and adjustment of the non-transitioning significant other. The gender actualizing individual needs strong support to help sort out the deep existential themes that will impact everything, even the relationship. The clarity achieved through affirming gender therapy will be needed for the reconstruction of the relationship house. For example, what does transition look like, and what's the intended outcome? What are the needs associated with gender actualizing that will impact the relationship? Attachment work will help the transitioning partner improve many relationship behaviors. This process is also necessary for the healing of the relationship because it allows the non-transitioning person to get to know the gender actualizing identity to gauge their own ideas about the relationship.

Framework for Transitioning Couples Therapy

Gender therapists working with transitioning couples should seek additional specialty in couples counseling. Before I heavily pursued my gender specialty, I had three years of training under by supervisor who is highly seasoned in couples therapy, niche in infidelity and high conflict; he is trained in Milan systemic and Satir approaches to couples work and passed knowledge to me. Much of my approach in transitioning couples is framed in the infidelity work I was trained in where we move the couple through three linear phases. The goal is to not move on to the next phase until the phase they are in is completed (like the card game Phase 10). The reason I compare transitioning couples work to infidelity work is not intended to induce shame or guilt on behalf of the transitioning partner. The reason is because the dynamics are incredibly similar at the core. When the core context a relationship is built on has ended, inevitable trauma occurs to the relationship foundation. For infidelity it's heavily the commitment contract that's violated, and for transitioning couples it also is rooted in that commitment but in a different way. The commitment contract, that occurs in a relationship before a partner comes out, is a promise of *who* you are committing to. For infidelity it is *what* you are committing to.

Phase 1: Addressing the Impact

During this phase, the clinician should address the impact of the disclosure of the trans person coming out for each partner personally and on the relationship. The therapist should teach and facilitate structured communication to guide couples through this process. Initially, this dialogue structure should be modeled in sessions so the couple can translate the steps at home. The clinician should openly recognize that both partners are hurting deeply at this time and prioritize creating an environment where both people are able to openly process their hurts together and in an effective way that promotes healing. Orchestrating the communication so that it nurtures the needs of both partners is a skill necessary in working with transitioning couples as the therapist attempts to unite them again. This is the stage for lots and lots of talking. This is also the time in treatment we formulate appropriate plans for stabilizing relational crisis which may include boundary setting, answering difficult questions, and creating a plan for supporting individual mental health needs.

The mental health provider will know it is time to move on to the next stage when the couple has reached a point in stabilization from crisis and both individuals inform the clinician, they feel heard, affirmed, and supported. This can be a vague concept to grasp since it looks different from every couple. My indication they are ready based on my own assessment is that all the needed talks have been had and the couple is pushing for more forward movement rather than processing the past or present hurts or responses to relational trauma. I will typically have a discussion with the couple, reflecting my own observations and impressions and asking for their ideas about readiness to move to the next stage.

Sometimes a difficult dynamic can present itself early in the therapy process, which is the couples' resistance and avoidance to approaching the gender actualization and transition needs of the trans person. This is quite common and honestly frustrating at times because it's hard not to feel stuck, in this locked dilemma, with the couple. For the transitioning partner, either retreating back to the closet or completely freezing is an automatic response to the trigger of a negative reaction to their authentic identity. The non-transitioning partner is stuck in a state of grief and is experiencing the exact same stages as transitioning families (stages mentioned in Chapter 9) in response to their significant other coming out. The stage I most commonly see the non-transitioning partner paused in is the *conditional accommodation* stage. In contrast to transitioning families, I notice the non-transitioning partner in a transitioning couple jump quickly through the first two phases to that one, and I suspect this has to do with the difference in power and role dynamic within the relationship. Because of the dangerous interaction between the grief response and the automatic response of retreat, the avoidance of movement can feel impossible at times for the clinician.

Clinical Example

Jess and Kara have been in weekly couples therapy for eight sessions with their therapist after Jess came out to Kara five months ago, informing her she is a trans woman and wants to transition. The couple has barely touched on this event in their sessions and often redirect therapist to other negative interactions within the relationship they could work on. Their progress has completely stagnated and hasn't moved much since the second session. Jess expressed in the first session she would ideally like to start HRT, get a new wardrobe, grow her hair out, and experiment with makeup to explore her gender expression. Kara was firm with Jess and therapist that she isn't ready for this yet.

There have been reports of conflict about Jess' desire to move forward in transition, but when the therapist attempts to engage the couple in discussion, Jess becomes passive and quiet and Kara continues to state she just isn't ready yet. Kara shared with counselor that she is using the name Jess and "allows" exploring clothes but has a hard line with makeup and HRT. Kara also states she isn't ready to use pronouns for Jess yet and that she isn't attracted to women so they will divorce if Jess transitions. There are three perceptions conflicting in this dynamic.

Jess is frustrated she cannot move forward in her transition but is too afraid to lose Kara. She feels resentful of the ultimatum. Jess has always put her gender identity on the back burner after she attempted to come out to her mother at age 12 and got a negative reaction. This is an automatic response for her, to retreat for the comfort of others. Jess feels like she has been able to live without her needs this long, and losing Kara is a perceived greater loss than transition because transition is a completely uncertain and ambiguous process. Would she even be happy on the other side? Is that risk worth losing the only person in her life she can be mostly herself with, her best friend? Jess also hopes Kara will come around on her own and doesn't want to push her out of fear of pushing Kara to leave.

Kara is completely devastated and doesn't know how to even begin unpacking her grief. She feels like her spouse is dying, and putting off addressing transition is keeping her spouse alive longer. Kara feels like if she and Jess can improve other aspects of their marriage and give Jess some flexibility to explore her trans identity, she might be able to protect and preserve their relationship. Kara doesn't understand trans identities and has only been exposed to trans people in the occasional television show. Kara has done some research to confirm her bias that trans people can change their minds. Maybe if she delays this, Jess won't need to transition when their relationship improves in other ways. Or maybe Jess needs to find happiness in herself in another way, maybe then she won't need to transition. Kara doesn't feel attracted to women and has decided if Jess transitions, this will mean divorce.

The perception of the therapist is feeling stuck with the couple. The clinician is aware that addressing Jess' gender identity and transition is the necessary next step for this couple to make any movement because it's at the core of their tension and negative interactions. The clinician notices that Kara is stuck in her grief process which is causing resistance in her behavior. The clinician also recognizes that Jess is taking a passive role to placate Kara, a common behavior with roots in anxious attachment and internalized stigma. Both Jess and Kara are refusing to take next steps to progress in the relationship and are avoiding the truth that there is absolutely no going back. This will continue to fester between them. In the meantime, Jess has relinquished her autonomy and choices about her transition to Kara so that she can ease her guilt and avoid impacting the relationship any further. Kara has assumed the role of control over the transition process as an adaptation of both Jess' lack of consistency and deferment of responsibility. Kara's lack of openness to Jess' needs and perception is rooted in her grief and desperation to preserve the relationship.

This is a common dynamic in transitioning couples work. It is important for the couples therapist to balance both a nurturing and transparent stance. In this case with Jess and Kara, I would take time in the early sessions to address both individuals and their current experiences with grief of the changing relationship. In this work process, I would coach the partner who is not doing the emotional work at the time with me to be an observer and reflect and be attentive to their significant other. If the couple isn't ready to address how the relationship is changing, I will slow it down and try to engage the couple together in some individual work to unite them as much as possible. Facilitated and structured dialogue is the most valuable and used tool for this stage. I would also be mindful of resistance and avoidance and challenge the couple with my transparent reflections about dynamics I am noticing, while engaging the couple to react and collaborate on how we make movement.

Phase 2: Changes in Context

This phase is typically the longest phase couples participate in. It's the stage where we analyze the vulnerabilities in the past and the present relationship and identify goals and areas of growth for the relationship. Especially with transitioning couples, developing closeness and intimacy is important to keep the couple united and exploring their new relationship. The work in this phase is incredibly important for the underlying decision-making process, which is a constant background question in transitioning couples work. Intimacy building interventions can be a variety of approaches, like facilitated dialogue, in-between session tasks designed to meet emotional needs and promote closeness, and experiential interventions in session to explore and connect the couple through self-actualization and growth.

This stage is complete when the couple is ready to decide and/or reports significant satisfaction in their relationship. That slowing down or lag starts when the couple is thriving on their own. Sometimes it's when the couple comes to me to express, they feel like they should end their relationship. Unfortunately, it's a coin-flip when it comes to the odds of transitioning couples continuing their relationship or breaking up. This is because that entire context changes, as the foundations that made the initial relationship are no longer there. For those that continue their relationship, there is potential for significant growth and closeness of the couple. It can be confusing during the decision-making process to identify differences between strong friendship intimacy and romantic intimacy, and it might help to structure dialogue around this experience and how it fits into the desire and wants for the future relationship.

If the couple decides to end their relationship, the clinician needs to assess their role and their comfort level with what comes next based on their own professional experience and practice. Personally, my approach is to not provide mediation services since I do not have training in this, and typically I refer out. There are times I will provide one or two termination sessions to help the couple engage effectively in discussions around their plans for separation and establishing supportive systems and resources. I have known couples to maintain friendships post separation and even successfully co-parent children in a way that keeps positive presence of both parents supporting custody. I will also refer both individuals for personal counseling if they want to use that resource so they can process the complexity of grief surrounding the ending of a relationship that ended very uniquely. Much of the time there is still profound love and admiration for one another, but lack of ability to connect within the next context in a way that supports a committed romantic relationship. It's important for the trans partner to continue their process of gender actualization and the non-transitioning person to process next steps for themselves.

Clinical Example

Michelle and Trish have decided to end their eight years of marriage. Trish is incredibly supportive of Michelle's gender actualization process as a trans-feminine person, and Michelle was very attentive to Trish while they moved forward in their transition. Michelle and Trish are incredibly close, and their friendship is the biggest strength in their marriage. Trish recognized that she has deep emotional love for her spouse, but her attraction to men is not as fluid as she has wished it to be. Michelle has found in their own process that they are growing and changing as a person and is open to ending the marriage because they don't know if their goals and needs align anymore with being married to Trish. Michelle also questions their own sexuality and growing attraction for men. As things wrap in therapy, the clinician facilitates some communication around processing the grief about the end of the relationship which the couple finds helpful. There are also some discussions about supporting one another and how each individual will organize their own resources and support during the divorce. The clinician provides a referral for mediation if it is needed.

Phase 3: Moving Forward

The new relationship house is almost done; it's time for analyzing and discussing what moving on from the old relationship looks like for the couple. This includes prevention work such as defining new boundaries for the couple. How will family and community be addressed? Sometimes a straight couple will now be perceived as a gay couple; how will the couple deal with this going forward? What support and resources can the couple engage in as they walk into the world differently? During this phase we make plans to encourage ongoing progress and healing beyond treatment. This stage is about a lot of logistical stuff and organizing plans for the future.

Clinical Example

Sara and Blake have done great in stabilizing their relationship since Blake came out prior to treatment eight months ago. Sara's hardest struggle was coping with her relationship changing from a lesbian dynamic to a straight one, as she found lots of affirmation and power in her lesbian identity. She found peace in the idea that she is still a lesbian and she is also in a straight relationship, and she is comfortable in the fluidity of her sexuality which didn't make her fear Blake's gender actualization process. Blake has felt mostly supported by Sara, even though there have been some bumps in the road and is doing personal therapy to support his gender actualization process.

The couple is currently working to improve overall relational satisfaction surrounding communication and conflict resolution, and they are making significant process. The couple feels ready to have Blake come out to their four- and six-year-old children. Sara is more concerned than Blake and has been struggling to commit to taking action. She is worried about how this change will impact the children, and Blake feels deprived of an opportunity to connect even more closely with his children by coming out and being open about his transition. Time is ticking because the children are starting to ask why Blake is growing facial hair and his voice sounds like he has a cold (he started HRT six months ago).

The therapist notices that Sara may be having a grief trigger. These triggers are normal as the couple rebuilds their relationship house around the new context. In addition to grief of her changing spouse, she might also be feeling grief regarding her own dreams of the future where she imagined raising her family in a household with two women. Sara also has valid concerns about the mental health of her children, especially if she is uninformed. The clinician will take time to affirm and validate her concerns and introduce some psychoeducation about how resilient and adaptable children are. The therapist will also explain risks and benefits, including the benefit that the children and Blake will be able to have a more secure attachment since the children will bond to the authentic Blake and not his performance. There are children's books to help normalize gender diversity, and the clinician will teach some tools to help Sara and Blake with this process as a united front.

The identity of the therapist should also be considered in transitioning couples work since it can present in the therapeutic relationship between couple and therapist. Cisgender clinicians should be acutely aware of the privileges of their gender identity and how it can impact a heightened feeling of vulnerability and lack of trust for the trans partner. A cis identifying therapist can also experience the non-transitioning partner's alignment with them. All identities that can lead to relating or aligning between partner and therapist should be considered; this is not an exclusive consideration for cis and straight therapists. Because of this inevitable countertransference, cisgender clinicians have a responsibility to not only be highly conscientious and mindful of their privilege's impact on their interactions in session, but actively address it. By modeling transparency around this dynamic, the intent is to increase comfort for the couple confronting or reflecting impact of the transference and countertransference being experienced.

Working with transitioning couples is a very specialized niche due to the incredibly unique and dividing experiences of both partners paired with the clinician's role of uniting them despite that opposition. Additional clinical experience is also required to be effective, as having a specialty in gender therapy is not enough. The orientation chosen for the approach to couples therapy isn't too important, as long as the clinician can be effective with it. I was trained from a Milan systemic oriented therapist but draw heavily from emotionally focused therapy (EFT). My past experience with infidelity work, which was a primary clientele I was trained in, has been highly useful for this task due to my comfort and familiarity in the trauma-response in the transitioning partner, feelings of guilt and shame in the partner disclosing relationship-altering information, and uniting a couple in a situation that feels emotionally dangerous to trust. In reverse, a couples therapist without training in gender therapy needs training to understand the special dynamics that is solely seen with transitioning couples only.

Reflection Questions for Clinicians

1   What is your process for stabilizing a relationship in crisis? If you do not have one, organize your process. How will you know stabilization has been achieved?
2   How would you respond to a dynamic where the non-transitioning partner is setting rules for the transitioning partner regarding what they are allowed to and not allowed to do in their transition?
3   How might aligning occur between therapist and partner? For example, if the therapist is cisgender and straight and the non-transitioning partner is also cis and straight, how might the aligning impact the therapy or interactions in sessions?

Index

For Product Safety Concerns and Information please contact our EU
representative GPSR@taylorandfrancis.com
Taylor & Francis Verlag GmbH, Kaufingerstraße 24, 80331 München, Germany

www.ingramcontent.com/pod-product-compliance
Lightning Source LLC
Chambersburg PA
CBHW060311220326
41598CB00027B/4297